Praise for *The*

MW01146323

In this beautiful book, my friend and fellow bishop Susan Goff chronicles her journey through the wilderness of breast cancer, from initial diagnosis to all the stages of treatment, all in the form of psalms, each one a poignant, honest outpouring of the heart. For any who find themselves entering that wilderness, here you will encounter a faithful companion and guide to the heart of a loving, liberating and life-giving God.

MICHAEL B. CURRY 27th Presiding Bishop of The Episcopal Church and author of *Love is the Way: Holding on to Hope in Troubling Times*

I usually read lying down on the couch or slouching in a soft chair. Before I finished the first two pages of this astonishing collection of psalms, I was either sitting bolt upright with my prayer beads, or literally kneeling at my prayer desk in my office. These are truly inspired. I know that because, though I have not faced cancer, I've faced other afflictions. Susan gave me words to pour out to God . . . And that's what psalmists, and true artists, do. [. . .] So much like the ancients, the setting and occasion of these urgent and eloquent psalms extend well beyond the person, place, and circumstances of Susan Goff's particular wilderness. The proof that the Spirit was at work in her compositions is that they will echo in the heart of anyone who is suddenly faced with the alarming diagnosis of being human. Anyone.

ROB HIRSCHFELD Episcopal Bishop of New Hampshire and author of *With Sighs Too Deep for Words: Grace and Depression*

In her beautiful book *The Desert Shall Rejoice: Psalms from the Wilderness of Breast Cancer*, Susan Goff walks alongside those going through cancer (and those journeying with them). A bishop in the Episcopal Church and a cancer survivor, Susan is a wise and compassionate companion for anyone walking cancer treatment's uneven path. Her psalms are honest and hopeful. You can trust her. She's been there. If you or someone you know is facing cancer, this book is an indispensable emotional and spiritual resource.

JAKE OWENSBY Episcopal Bishop of Western Louisiana and author of *Looking for God in Messy Places: A Book About Hope*

In this exquisite, unique treasure of a book, Bishop Susan Goff explores in poetry one of the most intimate of female experiences: breast cancer. As the biblical psalms express the full gamut of human emotions, so Bishop Susan describes her honest grief and fear, her vulnerability and her prayer-filled hopes, from the beginning discovery of a mass to her "cancerversary." She writes her poem-psalms with deep compassion and insight, playful humor, focus on God, and always great creativity. The vibrant, colorful book cover which she painted as a gifted artist, portrays the tender blossoming of the desert, even in the wilderness of breast cancer. I am deeply touched that a woman leader of the church would open up her life to us in this way. I highly recommend this book for anyone who has received a cancer diagnosis, for those supporting a family member or friend in the wilderness, and for clergy who want to understand something of this journey.

SARA PALMER Rector, All Souls Episcopal Church, Washington, DC

This book of psalms—prayers, laments, songs—not only tells the story of one woman's breast cancer journey; it reflects the reality that so many of us have gone through. This book is for those who us who have made this journey, for those who are in the middle of it, for those who find themselves starting down this path, and for the health professionals working with us. You will find affirmation, hope and love written in every psalm.

DIANE JARDINE BRUCE Bishop Provisional of the Episcopal Diocese of West Missouri and cancer survivor

With generous and blazing candor, Susan invites readers to her journey with cancer, but more, she beckons us to be curious, to be present, and to be honest. These psalms tell her story, and encourage us all to wonder what is real and what is possible. Whether experiencing anger or exhaustion, feeling "more and less alone than ever," noticing her body's fragility while being being grounded in the Body of Christ, seeing miracles in "the words of strangers," exploring perfectionism and permission, "crying [her]self out," or playing with words, humor, and colors, Susan's abundant sharing calls us to reflect on our own stories and to pour ourselves into the fullness of life in all its wild, stunning, and wide array.

MARTHA JONES BURFORD Community Builder and Musician, Grace Episcopal Church, Lexington, VA

the Desert Shall Rejoice

the
Desert
Shall
Rejoice

PSALMS
FROM THE
WILDERNESS
OF BREAST
CANCER

SUSAN E. GOFF

BOLD
STORY
PRESS

CHEVY CHASE, MARYLAND

Bold Story Press, Chevy Chase, MD 20815
www.boldstorypress.com

Copyright © 2024 by Susan E. Goff

All rights reserved. No part of this book may be reproduced or used in any manner without written permission of the copyright owner except for the use of quotations in a book review. Requests for permission or further information should be submitted through info@boldstorypress.com.

New Revised Standard Version Bible, copyright 1989, Division of Christian Education of the National Council of the Churches of Christ in the United States of America. Used by permission. All rights reserved worldwide.

This book is a memoir, and it reflects the author's present recollections of experiences over time.

Library of Congress Control Number: 2024920776

ISBN: 978-1-954805-66-8 (paperback)
ISBN: 978-1-954805-67-5 (e-book)

Cover painting by the author
Text and cover design by KP Books
Author photo by Susan Tilt

Printed in the United States of America
10   9   8   7   6   5   4   3   2   1

In memory of, and thanksgiving for, my mother,
Dorothy Goff. Even while dying of breast cancer,
she taught me how to live with
strength and courage, dignity and hope.
She was always ready for a journey.

Contents

A MONKEY WRENCH IN THE WORKS

ENTERING THE WILDERNESS

DISRUPTION

CHEMO BLUES AND OTHER COLORS

BALD!

JOURNEYING ON

COMING ALIVE

LOOKING BACK, LOOKING FORWARD

AFTERWARD

Preface

In the late winter of 2020, as the COVID-19 pandemic was beginning to rock our world, my world was further rocked by a diagnosis of invasive ductal carcinoma. Within a dozen days of my annual screening mammogram, I found myself among the twelve and a half percent of women who experience breast cancer in their lifetime. My husband joined the one out of every eight families who encounter breast cancer with a loved one. We became part of a club we never wanted to join, a society whose invitation we had never received and would never have accepted.

My first responses to the news that I had breast cancer were all over the place. I was in shock. I was in denial. I was annoyed, feeling that I just didn't have time for this. When I listened to my body, I knew that I was terrified. It made no sense at all that I had cancer, even given the high incidence of breast cancer in general and the high incidence of breast and related cancers in my family. My Aunt Jo died of breast cancer when I was a young adult. My mother, who had lived through the diagnosis and treatment of colon cancer, had a harder time with breast cancer, from which she died when she was in her nineties. My oldest sister, Dyanne, lived for fourteen years after her diagnosis of ovarian cancer and died of complications from the treatment, not from the disease itself. A cousin and two nieces went through breast cancer treatment and are doing well now. As I remembered those women and many others, my initial shock, fear, and annoyance were joined by curiosity and fierce determination. I chose to take on breast cancer treatment as a project. I made a decision not to battle breast cancer or become a cancer warrior, since I didn't want that violent imagery in my life at such a tender time. Instead, I chose the imagery of walking through the forbidding wilderness of breast cancer, intent on feeling what I was feeling and learning what I could about fear and hope, pain and patience, disruption and opportunity.

The psalms in this collection began as journal entries. I wrote every day, from the first call telling me that something suspicious showed up in my annual screening mammogram, through surgeries, chemotherapy, and radiation. I wrote to keep myself honest about my feelings, to process the journey, and to look for signs of hope in a new, surprising, and often dark landscape. After my final surgery, when I went back and read the journal from the beginning, I noticed that many entries were already like psalms in their form and in their unapologetic expression of emotions. With that recognition, I took on a discipline of shaping the raw material into poetry and sometimes song. As I shared early drafts of psalms with trusted friends and as I did readings of some of my favorites with small groups, I heard a range of responses. They included, "Me, too," and "Thank you for putting my experiences into words," and "Now I understand a little more about what my partner was going through." Those responses galvanized me to complete the psalms, bring them together in a book, and work with a publisher to put them into the hands of readers.

As I complete this manuscript, I am four years out from my initial diagnosis. I am doing well, though I'll admit that I can scarcely wait to complete five years on an aromatase inhibitor. I've made peace with the side effects of that medication for now but will be thrilled to be rid of them. In fact, I'll enjoy writing a psalm about dancing away from the little white pill and all the comfort-depleting yet life-giving effects it had on me.

It is my deepest hope that these psalms will support you on your journey through the wilderness of cancer, as you walk the way with a loved one, as you support women with breast cancer professionally, or as you continue to process your journey of years ago. I hope as well that, as you read my experiences, you will be strengthened to tell your own story boldly, honestly, and without apology. After all, fearsome journeys become a little less terrifying as we share them in words and images, tears and laughter, movement and poetry and song.

Introduction

In many traditions, psalms are poems or songs that express a community's relationship with the divine, however the community understands the divine. Psalms are packed with feeling, ranging from the deepest despair to the highest joy, from anger to thanksgiving, from lament to praise. The wilderness of breast cancer elicited in me every one of these feelings and more, making the psalm form perfect for telling this story.

While these psalms appear in the chronological order of my experience, they don't have to be read in order. Feel free to start at the beginning or to dive in with the psalm that calls out to you.

Most of these psalms are written in free verse and don't follow strict poetic rules. That means that there are no rules about how you are supposed to read them. You might try reading one or two out loud since, in most traditions, psalms are meant to be sung or recited. Pay attention to the words that call out to you, the experiences that echo your own, and those that are different from yours.

Pay attention as well to feelings. Let yourself feel what you are feeling as you read and as you reflect on your own journey. Well-meaning friends might be quick to tell you how you ought to react, how you should feel, and what emotions you should reject or ignore. Love them for trying, then feel what you are feeling no matter how raw, no matter how uncomfortable it makes them.

As a person of faith, I tell my story using language and imagery from the Bible and from *The Book of Common*

Prayer of The Episcopal Church, in which I am a bishop. As you reflect on and tell your story, dip into the language and imagery of your own spiritual or faith tradition, your favorite literature or movies, your family and community sagas—whatever sources give you the words you need to express your experience and to hold on to hope.

Citations for biblical passages that I quote in these psalms, all of which are from the New Revised Standard Version of the Bible or from the translation of the biblical Psalms in *The Book of Common Prayer*, are found in the Endnotes.

May my words be a support and grace to you as you travel your path and tell your story.

A Mass in My Breast

PSALM FOR
A Routine Screening Mammogram

Praise, O praise to you, God,
For the little gifts this day.

Praise to you, welcoming God,
For the kind woman who checks me in
and checks my history,
Who checks out my purple hair
and compares it with her own.

Praise to you, attentive God,
For the women in the waiting room,
each with her own story,
Some worried, some bored,
some ready to check the task off their list.

Praise to you, comforting God,
For a hot cup of tea in a tall paper cup,
And a toasty warm robe on a cold, cold morning.

Praise to you, empowering God,
For a mammographer who is kind and well-practiced
And tells me how her life is a '60s pop song.

Praise to you, discomfiting God,
For the press and squeeze of which I've always said,
"Better this momentary affliction than the long-term
affliction of cancer."

Praise to you, God who knows all,
That I'm done for another year.

PSALM FOR
A Callback

"I don't want this, O God.
I don't want any of this."
I cry these words in my dream
just before I wake at the crack of dawn,
terrified and in a cold sweat.
I don't want any of this, not today, not ever.

I received a callback yesterday.
A kind woman from the imaging center
said something showed up in my right breast.

I had a callback once before, six years ago.
I knew right from the start that it was nothing.
I was not afraid. I was not in denial. I just knew.
And it proved to be so.

This time is different. This time it feels real. Close.
Dark and murky. In a mirror dimly.
In a nightmare with Mom, who died of breast cancer.
In a dark dream where my seat and my stuff
are at the far corner of the table
and I am exhausted
and can scarcely stand upright
and can't begin to figure out
where I'll get the strength to take my seat.
In almost but not quite despair, I cry out,
"I don't want any of this,"
and wake up with a start.

I really don't want this, O God.
Not any of it.
I am afraid. Not that this will kill me,
but that it will disrupt everything,
that I'll lose every pretense of control,
that I'll—what? Feel like a failure?
That I won't be able to hide myself
in work and doing for others?

God, help me. God, stay with me.
Walk with me through this long week and weekend
until I go back for a second mammogram,
and maybe a sonogram,
and maybe news that will change my life.

The Callback Nightmare

Someone is carrying an infection,
someone is a monster threatening everyone.
We realize that we can tell who it is
by the coding on their name tag.
I go to the house I grew up in.
Mom is there. We run across the street.
I am wearing only panties and a short tee shirt,
but shrug my shoulders.
Mom says, "You know, Susan,
I'm going to have to check your name tag, too."
"Mom, you made my name tag; you know what's there!"
"I still have to check it."
"OK, I'll take it out when we get back home."
Impetuously I tease her,
"Maybe I'll have to check yours, too.
How do we know *you're* not the one?"

Then we stand before the door.
We open it.
It is pitch black inside.
We enter.
I hold the cold metal railing.
I hear a sound and whisper, "What's that?"
It sounds again. Louder. Closer.
Suddenly Mom is not my comfort.
Suddenly Mom is what I fear.
I wake from the nightmare.
Screaming. Terrified.

God help me. Save me from these night terrors.
Give me strength and courage.
Make this just one more false alarm.

PSALM ON
The Way to the
Callback Appointment

Jesus, I remember.
Jesus, I cling to what you have promised.
Jesus, I hold tight to what I preach in your name.
> I am light for the world.
> I am salt of the earth.
> I am loved.
> I am blessed.
> I am enough.

I can walk this road, because you walked it first,
> this road of fear,
> this road of suffering,
> this way of death that leads to life.

I can do this. I can deal with whatever comes this
morning.
> I am not weak because you are my strength.
> I am not (too) afraid because you are my comfort.
> I am not alone because you are with me.

Stay with me, strong Jesus.
Give me clarity to listen today.
Take away my fear
and let me embrace your love
more fully than ever.

The Callback Appointment

Gabriel, the messenger of peace,
Gabriel, the angel who brings good news,
Gabriel, whose words change everything,
does the ultrasound,
points to the image, and says,
"When it looks like this, it is virtually always cancer."
It looks so big on the screen.
"It's one centimeter," he says.
"It is deep inside.
It could not have been found in a self-exam.
The lymph nodes look fine."

It's easier now.
My courier of peace
spoke to me with clarity and calm.
He conveyed a message of truth,
this message that something has changed in me,
and I know that something, by God's grace,
might yet be born in me.

So, here's what I will paint—
a doctor in a white lab coat,
angel wings sewn where his name should be,
standing before a bare breasted woman
with the words "Do not be afraid"
swirling around them in myriad languages.

With that image and with those words,
I am not afraid. Today I am not afraid.

The Mass in My Breast

I picture the mass in my breast.
Not one that is
>chaotic
>and terrifying
>and growing

But a feast
>of bread and milk,
>of rich food filled with marrow,
>a land flowing with milk and honey.

This is my body that will bleed
>so that healing can be done.
This is my body that will break
>so that wholeness can be restored.
This is my scared and sacred body
>that will be scarred
>for the very life of me.

I do this in remembrance of you.

PSALM FOR
What Was Supposed to Be

I was supposed to be in Zanzibar this week
To meet with bishops from around the world.
I was supposed to be in Zanzibar this week,
A place that sounds exotic and so far away.
I was supposed to be in Zanzibar this week
With a quick side trip to Tanzania.
What a journey it would have been!
What adventures I might have had!

But I made the decision not to go
Before cancer reared its head.
I made the decision not to go
Last fall, before I knew.
I made the decision not to go
All for good reasons then . . .

. . . and now
It's clear I made exactly the right choice.
I chose then, unsuspecting, to make room for now,
For this journey that is unfolding,
For adventures I am having
In this strange and exotic land.

Thanks be to God for best-laid plans
And for my decision not to follow them,
For coincidence or intuition,
Fortuity or grace,
And the new ways the old pieces come together.
Thanks be to God for the grace of space.

PSALM FROM
The Biopsy

Just call me the Bionic Woman
with a titanium marker in my breast
placed there by a doctor with heart
after she took five samples from the tumor site,
each the size of a grain of rice.

"Close your eyes," she says after I am numb.
I do. Then I open them.
"What am I not supposed to see," I ask.
"Oh, you can see it," she replies,
"But most people don't want to."
"I want to see everything that is happening to my body."
(Is that really true?)
I look at the needle, a huge honking thing.
I watch on the screen as she inserts it,
not feeling even a pinch. She removes the samples
and places the titanium.

During the procedure we talk.
We note that each of us has lost
the accent of the place where we grew up.
We find a connection in the town
where I did my first chaplaincy.
She asks if I am still a chaplain.
I tell her I am a bishop.
We chat some more.
I comment on her competence and skill.
She says, "I can do this,

but I can't work a voice-activated TV.
My husband died last summer,"
she adds, seeming to surprise herself.
"I'm so sorry," I say.
"The little things really trip you up
when the big things are hard."
She then speaks with a technician and we say no more.
The silence is comfortable after shared vulnerability.

"Hallelujah, you're not a bleeder,"
she says when removing the needle.
My favorite mammographer,
whose name lights up a '60s pop song,
takes an image with light compression
to ensure that the titanium marker is in place. It is.
She gives me little round ice packs
to put inside my bra over the incision site.
"See you . . . " she hesitates. Then says too quickly,
"Next year. Not 'til next year, I hope."
"Thank you," I say. "I hope next year, too.
But if it's sooner, I'll be thankful you caught this early."

And off I go. The Bionic Woman. Titanium in my breast.
Ready for whatever comes.
God, make it so, please. Make it so.

Waiting for Biopsy Results

Friday night after the biopsy.
God, stay with me.

A long Saturday of normal activity.
God, stay with me.

A long Sunday of worship and prayer.
God, stay with me.

A long Monday, waiting for a call that never comes.
God, stay with me.

A long Tuesday morning and still no call.
I call everyone I can think of.
God, stay with me.

My primary care physician calls me back.
He tells me it is cancer.
He recommends a surgeon.
He assures me I'll be fine.
God, stay with me.

The radiologist who read the mammogram calls me back.
He apologizes for the delays.
He tells me it is cancer.
He gives me his cell number.
God, stay with me.

The radiologist who did the biopsy calls me back.
She tells me what I already know.
"I'm so sorry," she says, "This really sucks."
Her simple honesty helps.
God, stay with me.

God, stay with me as I take it in,
As I wonder, as I worry,
As I share the news.
God, just stay with me.
Because this sucks.
It really sucks.

The Pathology Report

Invasive Ductal Carcinoma
> Do not be afraid.
Grade 1
> Do not be afraid.
Not aggressive
> Do not be afraid.
One centimeter
> Do not be afraid.
No abnormal lymph nodes
> Do not be afraid.
HER2 negative
> Do not be afraid.
Progesterone negative
> Do not be afraid.
Estrogen positive
> Do not be afraid.
The cancer cells still have
some features of normal cells.
> Do not be afraid.
Next steps
An MRI
> Do not be afraid.
Surgery
> Do not be afraid.

Tonight, I am relieved.
Tonight, I can breathe.
Tonight, I am not afraid.
I am not too afraid.

Taking It In

PSALM OF
The Twelve and a Half Percent

I'd take those odds at a casino.
I'd play those odds on a lottery ticket.
I'd take a chance, a chance worth taking.

I didn't choose this game, though.
I didn't buy this ticket.
And yet, and yet

Since one out of every eight women
will have breast cancer in her lifetime,
then why not me?

Why, O why, God?
Why not me?

PSALM FROM
The Valley of the Shadows

"Though I walk through the valley
of the shadow of death,
I will fear no evil,
for you are with me.
Your rod and your staff,
they comfort me."

In the valley of shadows,
thick and murky,
I walk with confidence.

I carry my staff, my crozier,
down the aisle on Ash Wednesday
and I feel strength and comfort
as it keeps me steady,
keeps me grounded,
keeps me strong.

In the valley of the shadows,
your rod and staff hold me upright
and keep me going.

PSALM FOR
The Ashes

"Remember that you are dust
and to dust you shall return."

I say the ancient words
as I smear ashes onto foreheads
one day after receiving the biopsy report.

"Remember that you are dust
and to dust you shall return."

I remember, O God.
I wear my mortality on my forehead.

Surely they see it on my face
As I move along the communion rail.
Surely they see it on my face
As I see it on theirs.

The welcome mortality
        on the wizened faces
        of those preparing for death.
The burgeoning mortality
        on the resigned faces
        of those whose dreams are spent.
The veiled mortality
        on the open faces
        of those whose hopes run wild.

The alien mortality
    on the fresh faces
    of those who feel immortal.
The shocking mortality
    on the innocent faces
    of precious little children.

"Remember that you are dust
and to dust you shall return."

O yes, I remember, my God.
I remember as I wear this
    shocking
    alien
    veiled
    burgeoning
    not yet welcome mortality
on my ash-covered face.

Giving Up Fear for Lent

Every year when I was a child
I gave up chocolate for Lent.
I did it because my mother did.
My siblings did, too.

Sometimes we cheated
when the forty days began to feel
    like fifty
        sixty
            seventy
                a year
                    a lifetime.
Sometimes we cheated
and we still got chocolate bunnies for Easter.

Later I gave up TV
    that great time-sucker
        and read novels for fun
            instead of for English class.

Later still I gave up spontaneous spending
    dropping dollars for things
        I didn't need
            and hadn't planned for.

One year I gave up listening
    to the tapes in my head
        that tell me I'm not enough.
That one was particularly hard.
I've still not gotten the hang of it.

This year as I take up my mortality
I'm giving up fear.
You say to me, O God,
    through angels
        and prophets
            and friends
                and dreams,
"Do not be afraid."

This year as I wear my mortality on my face,
this year in the dust and ashes,
this year in the hope of Easter wonders,
I am giving up fear for Lent.

A Nurse Navigator

Oh God, you are my chart.
You are my compass,
my sounding line
and sextant.
You are the way ahead
who sent me a faithful navigator
to give me my bearings.

Two days after I got my biopsy results, she called me,
a woman in a position I'd never heard of before.

Two days after I got my biopsy results,
my nurse navigator called my cell phone
in the middle of a workday
and gave me seventy-five minutes of undivided attention.
An hour and a quarter she gave me,
  walking through every detail of the report,
  answering questions,
  offering hope,
  steering me,
  orienting me to strange new waters,
  and teaching me how to sail them.

Two days after I got my biopsy results, she called me
and told me about her role:
  to make connections between various doctors and
  offices,
  to make appointments for me,
  to give me the most up-to-date information.

Just two days after I got my biopsy results,
by George, I was blessed.

Oh God, you are my chart.
You are my compass,
my sounding line
and sextant.
You are the way ahead
who sent me a faithful navigator
to keep me on course.

PSALM FOR
When I'm Shaky

I am shaky, O God.
Literally.
I can't hold the pen
    to write inscriptions in the Bibles
    of those I will ordain on Saturday.
Literally.
I'm losing words,
my vocabulary is reduced to a five-year-old's.
My breath stops in my chest.
I have little appetite.

I am shaky, O God.
Literally.
I try to breathe deeply,
    in and out, in and out,
    and still I shake.

You say, "Do not be afraid"
And my body reveals that I am terrified.

God, give me rest.
God, give me breath.
God, calm my shaky,
    achy,
    breaky heart
And give me your peace.
I'm begging you.

PSALM OF
Meeting the Nurse Navigator

She came to the surgeon's office
just before my first appointment.
Although we'd never seen each other before,
    I recognized her instantly as soon as she walked in.
    Her spirit was lovely and alive.
She recognized me, too.
I introduced my husband, Tom.
We talked about cancer,
    about family,
    about life.
She gave me some booklets on breast cancer.
I felt known.
I felt supported.

I had no idea that it would be the only time
I'd see her without a mask.

PSALM AFTER
Meeting the Surgeon

I feel light,
almost giddy with relief.
The surgeon was kind,
    attentive,
    clear and caring.
He's had hundreds of meetings
    with hundreds of patients in his career,
    yet treated me as if I were the only one.
I spent two hours in his office,
    filling out papers,
    signing releases,
    asking questions,
    listening,
    learning,
    agreeing to genetic testing,
    saying yes to oncotype testing.
I see the plan before me,
    an MRI,
    a lumpectomy before the end of the month,
    three to six weeks of radiation.

I am giddy with relief.
I can do this!
Tom and I have lunch,
    in a restaurant on our way home,
    a precious midweek date.
    We plan to have lunch together

after every appointment
to treat ourselves
on the path ahead
now that the path is clear.
No more surprises.
We can do this.
With you, O God, we can do anything.

Spitting in a Vial

Praise God for spit.
Praise God for laughter.
Praise God for the genes
that have been passed down to me,
that make me who I am,
that connect me to family
across time and space.
Praise God for these genes.

The nurse practitioner in the surgeon's office
asks if I want to be tested for the
BRCA1 and BRCA2 mutations.
I ask many questions.
I get helpful answers.
I remember my mother,
 my great aunt,
 my cousin,
 and two nieces
 who had breast cancer,
 and my sister
 who had ovarian cancer.

I say yes.

She hands me a plastic vial
and tells me to spit to the fill line.
She leaves the room.

I begin.

I spit a few times and look at the vial.
Surely it is full.
It doesn't begin to measure.
I spit some more.
I think of lemons.
I think of Sour Patch candy.
I spit some more
    and some more
        and some more
and still, I'm so far from the fill line.

"I could do it in one spit," my husband says.
    (My dear husband who is with me
    for the last time before
    COVID restrictions exclude him.)
I bet he could.
Is it a gender thing?

I laugh and laugh and laugh out loud because I,
who can do so many creative and generative things,
    just can't seem to spit!

Finally, my spit reaches the line.
It's taken ten minutes.
The nurse practitioner returns.
I hand the vial to her, triumphant.
She looks and hands it back.
"It's got to be at or over the line, not just below."
She leaves and I spit again
    and again
        and again.

And I laugh again
    and again
       and again.
I could fill the vial more quickly with
tears of laughter than with spit.

Finally, finally, the vial is filled
    and I am emptied,
    emptied of pride
    and worry
    and a desire to control.
If I can't command my own spit,
what control do I think I have?

Praise God for spit.
Praise God for laughter.
Praise God for the genes
that have been passed down to me,
that make me who I am,
that connect me to family
across time and space.
Praise God for these genes.

PSALM OF
The Lovely Notes

People send me get-well cards.
They send me messages of strength and support
at the special email address we've set up.
They respond with words of encouragement
on the blog page I've begun.

The notes are lovely and heartfelt.
None sound perfunctory.
None feel obligatory.
They are truly loving—
and I can read only a few at a time.

Because the words,
often beginning with "I'm so sorry,"
don't fit my experience,
don't fit my self-image.

I'm not sick.
I don't feel sick.
I don't know how to be sick.
Except for the cancer, I'm fine.
Except for the cancer, I'm well.
Except for the cancer.

Maybe I'm in denial—
not about having cancer,
but about this being a thing,
a real thing,
a big thing.

I am fine.
Except for the cancer, I am fine.
I really am.

I read the notes only a few at a time
to let the reality sink in slowly.

The Kitchen Tools

I ask my surgeon, half in jest,
if he does the lumpectomy with
something like an apple corer.
He says many women ask that,
(I'm not as witty as I thought)
but it's more like a melon baller.
I picture the soft, ripe fruit
with its malignant blemish
and know I'll never think
of one ordinary kitchen tool
in the same way again.

First Tears

I read the booklets my
nurse navigator gave me.
So many steps yet to go.
So much lies ahead.
I feel overwhelmed.
For the first time
I go to bed and cry.

God, I didn't choose this.
God, I don't want this.
Yes, I know I can do it.
Yes, I know you are with me.
Yes, I know I am not alone.
And I still don't want it.

But since the only way out is through,
let's do it.
Let's do this thing.
God, let's do it.
Starting tomorrow, please.
For tonight, just let me cry.

Let the Healing Begin

PSALM OF
The MRI

Click Click Click Click
Whir Whir Whir
Beep Beep Beep Clang
Bang

Clang Clang
Whir Whir Whir Click
Beep Beep Whir Whir
Bang

Click Click Click Click
Whir Whir Beep
Clang Bang

Bang Bang
Beep Beep Click
Whir Whir Whir Whir
Bang

You're doing great.

Beep Whir Whir Whir
Click Click Beep Bang
Whir Whir Whir

Beep Bang Click
Click Click Bang Whir Whir
Whir Whir Whir Beep
Beep Beep Clang Click Bang

Almost done.

Whir Whir Whir Whir Whir Whir Whir
Click Beep Bang Click
Beep Clang Bang Click
Whir Whir Whir Whir Whiiiiiiiiiiiir

That's it. You did great!

PSALM FOR
Learning to Dye

The week before the mammogram,
I decided to learn how to dye
silk scarves with bleeding tissue paper
of the deepest blues and purples,
rose and orange and green.

I tore the paper,
     placed it,
          spritzed it with water,
and waited to see the beauty in living color.

It was not until the diagnosis was confirmed
that I realized what I had done.

Praise be to God for double meanings
     that bring laughter,
          that bring hope,
               that reveal the soul's inner work
long before I knew it had begun.

The Results of Genetic Testing

"You don't have the genetic mutations,"
 the nurse practitioner tells me.
"Not BRCA 1 or BRCA 2.
 We don't know why you got breast cancer;
 Of course, we rarely do."

Would it help if I knew?
Would it help if I could blame it on genetics?
Would it help if I smoked or drank or took drugs?
They don't know why,
 and I find I don't need to know.
There is a mass in my breast
 and I don't need to know why.
I'm just ready for it to be gone.

Thank you, God,
 for the marvels of medicine that tell us so much
—and so little.
Thank you, God,
 for the knowing
—and the not knowing
 and for being comfortable
 either way.

Waiting for Surgery

The date of surgery is set.
Just ten days away.
And every day this new virus
threatens everything.

Tents appear in the hospital parking lot.
The emergency room is full.
Elective surgeries are canceled.

So far, a lumpectomy is not considered elective.
Will that change in the next week and a half?
Will I be bumped for more immediate needs?

What about the women
who have not had their mammograms?
Will they be bumped,
> their appointments put off,
> small tumors like mine
> left undiscovered
> until it is too late?

I see fear in the eyes of the medical personnel I meet.
They are kind,
> professional,
> responsive.
And afraid.

I suspend all worship
    in our churches and chapels for two weeks
    for the sake of the most vulnerable,
    for the protection of our healthcare system.
I write and send out
    statements,
    theological reflections,
    messages of hope.
I confer with colleagues,
    with my staff,
    with medical professionals.
I am exhausted and strangely exhilarated.
No wonder I collapse into bed
and sleep long hours.

I have two jobs right now, as I see it,
    to manage the anxiety
    in our stressed church system
    and to take care of myself
    so that I can have this surgery.

I take good care.
    And I wait.
        And wait.
            And wait.
Praying that
    my surgeon will stay well.
Praying that
    I will stay well.
Praying that
    the surgery will happen.

The Pre-op Appointment

This hospital feels like a ghost town,
eerily quiet, preternaturally still,
    no one in the halls,
    no announcements over the speakers,
    no newspapers piled on counters,
    no brochures in the racks.
Hand sanitizer bottles are the only sign
    that people might be near.
I am disoriented by the absences.

I entered through the emergency room.
A compassionate woman asked questions—
    have you had a fever or cough
    in the last fourteen days?
    have you traveled outside the county
    in the past two weeks?
    have you been in contact with anyone
    who has been diagnosed with COVID-19?

In the pre-op exam room,
    I answer more questions,
    blood is drawn,
    I am given instructions.
Everyone is kind.
And guarded.
It's like the throbbing stillness
    in a 1960s horror movie
    just before the violins screech
    and the monsters attack.

As I leave,
     the woman who asked the questions
     at the door tells me the news.
     As of this very hour,
     visitors may no longer enter the hospital.
     Tom will not be able to be with me
     on the day of surgery.
     I must walk in alone.

I am sad.
I am worried.
I am angry.
And I am grateful that
the surgery is still scheduled.
I am ready to get on with it.
I've paid the copay,
so I can't be bumped now,
right?

Ever-present God, you were there
     in the absence,
     in the weird hollowness,
     in the eerie silence.
Stay with me now.

PSALM FOR
The Night Before Surgery

As I make my bed again
with newly washed sheets,
As I fast from food and water,
As I shower with surgical soap,
then dress in absolutely clean pajamas,

I am a vestal virgin preparing for the sacrifice,
a bride preparing for her groom,
a performer preparing for opening night,
a traveler preparing for the journey.

In the morning, I will walk in alone.
I will strip naked before strangers
who will put me to sleep and cut my body.
I will put my life in their hands. Literally.
I will have no control.
I will wear no symbols to show who I am,
     no wedding ring,
     no bishop's ring,
     no cross.
Just the purple hair
And a plastic hospital bracelet.

Can I trust so deeply?
Can I surrender so fully?

As I prepare to place my life
in the hands of a medical team,
I surrender to you, O God.

And I choose
    to walk into the hospital tomorrow
    with grace and courage,
    to treat everyone I meet with kindness,
    to ask questions,
    to breathe,
    to let go of fear,
    to hold on to hope,
    to walk in love
knowing that I am loved,
knowing that I am not alone.

PSALM OF
The Surgery

Tom drives me to the hospital
and drops me off in the parking lot
of the cancer institute.
I kiss him goodbye,
>   put on a brave face,
>   put my mask over it,
>   and walk into the center
>   completely alone.
This just isn't right.
I remind myself to keep breathing.

They take my temperature
>   at the door for the first time,
>   the newest COVID protocol.
This just isn't right.
I remind myself to keep breathing.

A radiologist inserts a wire
from the top of my breast
>   to the titanium marker.
>   The procedure is awkward
>   but not painful.
>   I watch as much of it as I can,
>   all alone.
This just isn't right.
I remind myself to keep breathing.

I walk my newly wired and all-alone self
from the cancer institute,
    across the ER parking lot
    that is now full of tents
    for COVID testing
    and refrigerated trucks that I pretend not to see,
    to the main hospital building.
This just isn't right.
I remind myself to keep breathing.

I undress and put on a hospital gown.
A nurse tells me that I should leave my phone
    with my companion—
    and then she remembers.
    She puts it in the locker with my clothes.
This just isn't right.
I remind myself to keep breathing.

I overhear nurses at their station
    talking about a new regulation
    that no surgery may proceed
    without a signed statement
    by the surgeon
    saying that it is medically necessary.
This just isn't right.
I remind myself to keep breathing.

Someone from nuclear medicine
injects dye into my breast.
    I ask her if it will turn my hair purple.
    She laughs.
    Instead, it turns my pee electric turquoise.
This just isn't right, but it is funny.
My laughter keeps me breathing.

The IV is in. My contacts are out.
It's starting to feel like what I expected.
I can breathe.

My surgeon shows me images
of the wire in my breast.
He describes circumstances
in which I would need more surgery.
I'm not thinking about that now.
I keep breathing.

The nurse anesthetist injects
a sedative in my IV line.
It knocks me right out.
My body knows what to do.
I'm more alone and less alone than ever.
I don't have to remember to breathe.

PSALM FOR
Waking Up in Post-op

I wake up thinking I am at home in bed.
But there is a curtain at the foot of the bed
    and a stranger in forest green scrubs
    sitting at a desk with his back to me.
I try to ask him where I am, but my throat is dry.
Then I remember.

I feel awful,
    woozy, dizzy,
    groggy, sick.
They move me to a cubicle
    where the same day nurse tells me
    to get up and get dressed.
The room is rolling like old movie film
    that is off track in the projector.
    Breathing makes me nauseous.
I never want surgery again.

Tom is in the parking lot.
He's been waiting a while.
    He left the lights on
    and the key in the ignition.
When I'm finally ready for discharge
    the car won't start.
    Someone from hospital security
    gives the car a jump start.
An angel in disguise.

Home at last. In bed.
Mild pulling
and burning sensations
in my breast.
No pain at all.
    I feel awful.
    I feel vulnerable.
    I feel grateful.
    I feel supported.
    I keep breathing.
    And breathing.
    And breathing
until at last, I sleep in your loving arms, O God.
Until at last, I breathe deeply and sleep.

The Pathology Report

My surgeon calls a week after surgery.
Wonderful news.
Margins are clear.
Lymph nodes are clear.
Hallelujah!
No more surgery!

With this news, I am flying high.
On to radiation!
On to the last leg of the journey!
Let the healing continue!

PSALM OF
Praise for Signs of Healing

Praise to you, O God,
for the itching,
prickling, tingling,
sweet, sweet sting
of a thousand ants
on my breast.

Praise to you, O God,
for the greenish yellows
and blues of bruises,
a confusion
of contusions
on my chest.

Praise to you, O God,
for the pulling off,
peeling up,
lifting curling edge
of liquid bandage
on my breast.

Praise to you, O God,
for all the signs of healing.
Praise to you
for all the signs of grace.

The Odd Couple

Cancer and coronavirus are an odd, unhappy couple.
Contrary, stubborn, cantankerous, cruel.
They pit themselves against each other
and vie for my attention.
Once one has got it, the other rips it away.

Cancer and coronavirus are an odd, unhappy couple.
Bull-headed, ornery, perverse, mulish.
They each demand the full command
of a house that was built for one.
Once they've moved in, there's room for nothing else.

Cancer and coronavirus are an odd, unhappy couple.
And I am sick and tired of them.
God, I'm sick and tired of them.

A Monkey Wrench in the Works

The Monkey Wrench

Now comes the monkey wrench thrown in the works.
Now comes the fly in the ointment,
 the bolt from the blue,
 the bombshell,
 the strike-me-dead-in-my-tracks
 and render-me-speechless news.

My nurse navigator calls with a game-changing update.
The genomic testing scores are in, she says.
The oncotype recurrence scores are in.
 They show, God help me,
 a high likelihood that
 this cancer will come back, God help me,
 within nine years, God help me,
 in liver, lungs or bones, God help me.
The scores show, God help me,
 a benefit from chemotherapy.
The scores suggest, God help me,
 a new road ahead.

Now there is a monkey in the ointment,
 a fly in the bolt,
 a blue in the bombshell.
I feel flattened as if by—oh, you know,
 one of those trucks
 with the roller thing on front
 that levels everything.

I'm OK, God help me, I am.
I'll be OK, God help me, I will.
But, come on, now! Come on!

PSALM
When I'm Angry at My Oncologist

O my God,
my oncologist is telling me things I don't want to hear.
She says high chance of recurrence
when I'm ready to be done.
She says chemo, chemo, chemo
when I want none of it,
and a port when I say no more surgery, ever.
Damnable oncologist.

How dare she!
How dare she keep interrupting my plans
with her reality!
How dare she tell me these things
    when no one can hear them with me,
    when I can't even see her face!
I am so angry,
    so angry that it is hard for me to hear her,
    so angry that it is hard for me to believe her,
    so angry that it is hard for me to trust her.
So angry as I work so hard not to let her see it
because none of this is her fault.

God, help me.
Take this anger that feels like
    a red-hot iron on my shoulders,
    a clamp on my heart,
    a lump in my breast.

I'm trying to lift it up to you, God,
    trying to get my hands under it to give it a shove,
    and it's just too heavy.

Take this fury away from me so that I can
    see what I need to see,
    hear what I need to hear,
    know what I need to know,
    do what I need to do,
and recognize the power of your healing grace
in the eyes and hands and voice
    of a masked and damnable oncologist
    who is just trying to do her best for me.

PSALM FOR
A Second Opinion

"You'll do fine during treatment,"
my radiation oncologist tells me.
Because the tumor was one centimeter,
the margins were clear,
and lymph nodes were not involved,
the shortest radiation protocol is recommended—
sixteen sessions, three weeks and a day.
I can do that!

"But you're wondering what to do about chemo."
Yes, O yes. Help me listen now, God.
Yes, O yes. Help me hear.

She explains that a recurrence rate
of eighteen percent is high.
She explains that the benefit of chemo
is absolute, not relative.
She explains that chemo would precede radiation.
She tells me the same things
my medical oncologist has already told me,
but this time, no longer in shock and anger, I can hear.
This time I can almost understand.

"If you had these numbers," I ask,
"Would you have chemo?"
Without a moment's hesitation, she answers:
"With all I've seen in this office,

all the metastatic breast cancer,
I'd do chemo in a heartbeat."
Her eyes tell me it is true.

I get up to leave and say,
"I'll see you—probably later than sooner."
"I think that is a wise choice," she responds.

God, I don't want this.
I don't want any of this.
I feel more comfortable now,
more confident now,
and I don't want this at all.

Help me listen. Help me trust.
Help me make this terrible
and terrifying decision.

PSALM FOR
A Third Opinion

This time the appointment
is with an out-of-town oncologist.
This time it is on my phone.
This time I can see her face!
All of her face!

She says I'll be able to work during chemo.
She says that some days I won't be at my best.
She says I will lose my hair and experience fatigue.
She says, "If this cancer comes back, I can't cure you."
She says, "People depend on you.
You want to be there for them."

She cuts right through to me.
"You want to be there for them."

PSALM FOR
Making the Decision

I sit on the back porch with Tom on a beautiful
 spring day.
"Eighteen percent doesn't sound so high," I say to him.
"But an almost one-out-of-five chance of recurrence does."

"It's kind of like Russian roulette," Tom says.
"If there were a gun with five chambers and a bullet in one,
 would you put it to your head and pull the trigger?"

"*Hell no!*"

Case made.
I don't want to do this.
It sucks, God.
I am anxious.
I hate it.
And I am doing it.

A Fourth Opinion

I'm not one hundred percent confident, O God,
I don't know that I ever will be.

But I've made a decision,
a yes to chemotherapy.

I call the office of the fourth oncologist
And cancel the appointment.

PSALM OF
Risks Versus Benefits

Over and over again,
it's about risks versus benefits.

The risk of side effects
    versus intended outcomes.
The risk of long-term consequences
    versus immediate relief.
The risk of potential peril
    versus probable gain.

Over and over again,
it's about risks versus benefits.

I read and read and read.
I ask questions and listen carefully.
I read some more.
I weigh the benefits.
I weigh the risks
    as if placing each
    on an old-fashioned scale.
(If only it were that easy.)

I tune in to my body's own wisdom
    and instincts
    and mounting experience

Until finally all I can do is take a leap
    and say yes to surgery,
    yes to testing,
    yes to chemo,
    yes to meds,
Then weigh it all again when the leap
takes me where I don't want to go.

PSALM FOR
A New Image

My best friend sends me a gift.
A small wooden box with a slide top.
A bracelet inside.
Tiny silver beads, some round, some oblong,
Dots and dashes of Morse Code
Spelling out FUCK CANCER.

I howl with laughter,
Feeling known and loved and prayed for
By my friend who knows breast cancer herself.
I laugh my utter delight until
Tears of gratefulness wet my cheeks.

But I don't want to fuck cancer.
I don't want that anger in my life.
I don't want to fight cancer or battle cancer
Or crush cancer or be a cancer warrior.
I don't want that violence in my life.

I take the bracelet apart and,
Following a Morse Code chart online,
Reconfigure the beads to say G'BYE CANCER.
I restring the bracelet with small stones
In rose and purple
And wear it to every appointment,
Every treatment, every infusion.

Instead of fucking or fighting,
I choose walking.
Walking in the wilderness of cancer.
Walking from fear back to hope,
From illness to health,
From worry to trust.
I chose to walk the wilderness road,
Determined to find the wonders there.

God, you gave manna in the wilderness,
Quails in the desert,
Water from the rock.
You loved your ornery people
through their wilderness wandering.
Love ornery me now, through mine.

Entering the Wilderness

The God of Numbers

I don't much like the god of the book of Numbers.
That god is petulant, immature, reactive, arbitrary.
That god is no more together,
>   no more grown up,
>   than the ornery
>   wilderness wanderers
>   who cry out to him.

I think of *Who Framed Roger Rabbit*, the 1980s movie.
Voluptuous cartoon figure, Jessica,
when caught in a web of jealousy and murder, explains,
"I'm not bad; I'm just drawn that way."
Maybe the god in Numbers is not petulant,
but just written that way.

That better be the case, O God,
because if I'm stepping into the wilderness with you,
I don't need petulant. I don't need arbitrary.
Cancer has that territory covered.
Inscrutability I can take. Unpredictability I can embrace
(after all, I want more than I can imagine right now).
But let's leave that Numbers shtick behind.
I'll try not to act like a spoiled and entitled
wanderer in the wilderness
if you'll be the God whom Jesus loved,
the God who is pure Love.

The Cancer Patient

I am a cancer patient, O God.
Me, a cancer patient.
And that is shocking my world!

I'm not afraid that I'll die of this cancer.
That fear is not on the horizon.
I am afraid of being sick and fatigued.
I am afraid of going back to the hospital
    over and over again
    during a pandemic
    when there's so much illness there.
I am afraid of going to appointments alone
    with no one else to listen
    and take notes
    and ask questions.

I can do this.
That's not just pep talk language.
I am resilient and able to advocate for myself
and get the answers I need
(if only I knew the questions!)

I can do this.
I can do all things
through Christ who
strengthens me.
I just don't want to.

I am a cancer patient, O God.
Me, a cancer patient.
And that is shocking
    rocking
    blocking
    knocking
    mocking
    maybe even clocking
 my world!

PSALM OF
Feeling Betrayed

I dream disturbing dreams, O God.
You speak to me in dreams.

I am at the house I grew up in,
though it doesn't look like it at all.
I climb a long, long staircase at the back of the house,
moving up from the wild forest floor. It is dark.
By the time I reach the door, I am tired.

A woman I don't know, but who is vaguely familiar,
climbs the steps behind me.
Dyed blonde hair. Rough around the edges.
I don't see her in the house as I explore
the beautiful renovations of the kitchen and bathrooms.
I feel sad that Mom never got to see the changes.
Suddenly Mom is there. I realize I was confused,
that she's been there all along.

I prepare to leave through the basement door.
I see the blonde woman passed out on the bathroom floor,
urine and blood and drug paraphernalia all around her.
She is still a stranger and familiar, both at once.
I light into her.
"You have betrayed me.
I can't believe you did this here, in this house!
What is wrong with you?"

Even as I rant, I realize that I am not helping matters.
She is a human being, a child of God in trouble.

I start to wonder what I need to do in this situation.
She is so ill that she can do nothing.
"What would love do?" I wonder out loud.
I wake up to the sound of my own voice.

I've been angry and feeling betrayed by my own body.
I've been tempted to cuss it out.
Others encourage me to cuss cancer and fight cancer.
And none of that works for me.

I am the woman suffering on the bathroom floor.
And I am the woman asking, "What would love do?"

PSALM OF
The Port

On the morning of the day the portacath is placed,
The *Third Song of Isaiah* comes up in Morning Prayer.
"Arise, shine, for your light has come
and the glory of the Lord has dawned upon you.
For behold, darkness covers the land;
deep gloom enshrouds the peoples.
But over you the Lord will rise,
and his glory will appear upon you . . .
Violence will no more be heard in your land,
ruin or destruction within your borders.
You will call your walls, Salvation,
and all your portals, Praise."

And I know what I will call my port when it is placed.
I know what kind of prayers I will pray
each time the port is accessed.
Maybe when this is all over
I will have it tattooed on my chest,
right over the scars.
PRAISE.

PSALM OF
God's Silence

Once more, I can't settle down to pray.
The fears and decisions just keep spinning.
I turn to the recording of an anthem I have sung
with the House of Bishops choir,
its text first written on a cellar wall
by a nameless prisoner
in a concentration camp in Cologne, Germany.
> *I believe in the sun even when it's not shining.*
> *I believe in love even when I don't feel it.*
> *I believe in God even when God is silent.*

As I listen, the flood gates open.
I crumble in tears as I knew I would
when I chose the piece
(or when it chose me).
I cry in my prayer chair,
a worried pup in my lap.
I go into the hall and find Tom
and cry as he holds me.
We go into the bedroom
and lie down together.
He holds me even tighter
as I cry myself out.

The cry is exhausting.
Stress and fear and loss
and anger are exhausting.
Hearing God's silence

in answer to my questions,
not being able to pray for myself,
not feeling God's presence—
it is all exhausting.

I know this is not for all time.
I know it is a stage of the journey.
I know it is not unique to me.
I know that even when I can't pray for myself,
others are praying for me,
that the Spirit intercedes for me
with sighs too deep for words—
but I don't know it all right now.

Keep on interceding for me, Spirit.
Let me see the blessings,
the healing, the strength,
even in my weakness,
especially in my weakness.
Let me believe in you
even when you are silent.

The Port Placement

I go to Interventional Radiology to have my portacath placed.
>Praise be.

It is quicker and maybe safer there during a pandemic.
>Praise be.

The surgeon shows me the portacath.
>Praise be.

It's purple, like my hair, like the shoes I don't have to take off.
>Praise be.

It has a long, long tail.
>Praise be.

The whole long tail will not be needed, he'll cut off the excess.
>Praise be.

I'm given a local anesthetic and mild sedation.
>Praise be.

I cannot see what the team is doing, but I hear everything.
>Praise be.

I feel only pressure. I don't fall asleep.
>Praise be.

The doctor talks of the pizza he cooked on the grill last night.
>Praise be.

Others share their favorite pizza recipes.
>Praise be.

It all sounds delicious. My stomach rumbles.
>Praise be.

Please, can we change the subject?
I haven't eaten since yesterday.
>Praise be.

And they are done.
And I see on the screen the port in my chest
with its catheter to the superior vena cava.
    Praise be.
All ported up with somewhere to go.

PSALM OF
The Wilderness Walk

Off I go.
Into the wilderness.
Off I go to travel the unmarked path
    from the old normal of what was
    to the new normal of what will be,
a journey through complaints and regrets,
    rebellion and backward glances,
    discomfort, annoyance and uncertainty,
through wonders of manna and quails
    and water from the rock.
I don't want this journey, but I have chosen it.
I could have said no. I still can.
I don't think I will.

Instead, I will cooperate with my team,
    with my meds,
    with my Jesus,
    with myself.
I am not a victim.
I am a cooperator,
    a collaborator,
    a conspirer
    for my own healing.

"Be strong and courageous;
do not be frightened or dismayed,
for the Lord your God is with you
wherever you go."

Off I go.
Into the wilderness.

The Beautiful Gifts

My cousin sends me gifts she sewed;
    a soft pillowcase with messages of hope—
    courage, cure, love, believe—
    and a tote with images of bald or turbaned women
    for carrying my gear to infusions.
My cousin has taken her own walk
    through the wilderness of breast cancer.
    She knows.

Some nieces and nephews send me a box
    of colors, scents and love—
    a soft scarf, some fuzzy socks,
    a coloring book and lollipops—
    "Aunt Susan, we love you!
    Stay #SusanStrong!"
One of these nieces has taken her own walk
    through the wilderness of breast cancer.
    She knows.

Students from a campus ministry hold a virtual walk
    for breast cancer awareness.
    They send me photos of luminaries they made,
    one with a pink ribboned miter and the words,
    "#SusanStrong. We ♥ you."
The chaplain has taken her own walk
    through the wilderness of breast cancer.
    She knows.

A clergy couple of the diocese sends me the gift
        of light organic meals—
        bowls and flatbreads and soups
        to pack in the freezer and pull out when I need them.
Each of their mothers is taking her own walk
        through the wilderness of illness.
        They know.

The Diocesan staff holds an online hat party
        before my hair falls out,
        modeling what I should wear when I'm bald.
        They hijack a staff meeting with "Goat to Meeting,"
        a virtual visit with pigs and sheep,
        a llama and, of course, a goat.
We have taken our own walk
        through another wilderness together.
        They know.

Thank you, God, for the beautiful gifts
of your knowing and beautiful people.
Thank you, God, for the beautiful gifts
that touch and move me to tears.
Thank you, God, for the beautiful gift
that your people are to me.

The Cancer Cards

I create for myself some cancer cards before my first infusion,
a complete deck of fifty-two, each with an image
and a C-word to counter, contrast with and carp about
the other C-word in my life.
I'll play the cards cleverly on my own
and convey some to companions along the way.

I'll carefully play the cards that complain.
>Chemo sucks.
>Watch out, I'm crabby today.
>Chemo brane iz reel.
>The waiting makes me crazy.

I'll cheerfully play the cards that encourage.
>Never captive to cancer.
>Clear and present hope.
>Going for the cure.
>Change can be my friend.

I'll daringly play the cards that compel.
>Be of good courage.
>Cooperate.
>Cover yourself in glory.
>Choose life.

I'll creatively play the cards that console.
Not a catastrophe.
I can, but maybe not right now.
Keep calm and carry on.
Centered.

I'll compassionately play the cards that connect.
In good company.
We are one community.
Consult others.
I've joined the club.

I'll cackle as I play the wild cards.
Chocolate!
Crone-bound.
Crack me up, crack me open.
Bald is cute.

I'll clasp the jokers close to my breast.
Crap, crap, crappity crap.
Cantankerous, crotchety, cranky and cross.

Through it all, I'll stay centered
as I remember the context in confidence,
counting the days, avoiding clichés
and holding tight to the cross.

I create for myself some cancer cards to help me keep it real.

Disruption

PSALM OF
Holy Grieving

Grief is a new and constant companion.
Grief walks with me day after day
    and sleeps with me night after night.
And not only on this Good, but not so great, Friday.
Grief for those who are ill
    and those who have died
    in a pandemic that some falsely claim is a hoax.
Grief for the widening political breach in our nation
    that the coronavirus illuminates.
Grief that we can't worship in old familiar ways
    as we choose to protect the most vulnerable.
Grief when the decisions I convey
    and the guidelines I establish
    are met with vitriol and wild imputing of motives—
        communist,
        unGodly,
        unAmerican,
        selfish,
        cowardly,
        power-hungry.
Grief over those who say they love God
while erupting in vicious rage.

I say I don't let their rage in. But I do.
I say that I am not stung by the attacks. But I am.

I grieve the brokenness of the church.
I grieve the brokenness of our nation.
I grieve the brokenness of my own body
    even as it so miraculously heals.

I grieve. I mourn. I sorrow.
And not only on this Good, but not so great, Friday.
Grief is my constant companion,
drawing me close to the beating, broken heart of God.

Let me dwell there
    next to your heart
    for a time, O God.
Keep me safe there
    in the shadow of your love.
Make my grief a gift of healing
    from which I will never turn away,
    from which I will not flee.

PSALM OF
Holy Disruption

God, you act decisively through disruption.

You disrupted the chaos of roiling water and deepest darkness
    to create the world.
You disrupted the status quo of oppressed and oppressor
    to free the slaves of Egypt.
You disrupted the ordinary life of a teenage girl
    to birth love incarnate in the world.
You disrupted and destroyed the finality of death
    to bring life and immortality to light.

Now our lives are disrupted
    by the novel coronavirus.
Now our lives are disrupted
    by political divisions.
Now my life is disrupted
    by cancer and its treatment.

And you are present, God.
You, O God, are present.

What will I do in this time for which I will be grateful
when the season of disruption is over?
What will I lose in this time that I will ultimately
be grateful that I lost?

For now, I am curiously grateful for
    masks and physical distancing and staying home
    because they mean that I can work without fear
    during cancer treatment.

I am grateful for electronics and for Zoom
      because they mean that I can work in safety
      during cancer treatment.

God, keep me open to disruption in my life.
Let me see in every disruption an opportunity
to love you and serve your people.
God, let me embrace disruption for the sake of life.

PSALM OF
Being Prayed For

I walk a high wire. I've never done this before.
I should be terrified. I don't like these heights
when I'm so trembly that it's hard to keep my balance.
Yet I am, at times, surprisingly calm.

The prayers that people pray for me
are the long pole I hold for balance
and the net that is just three feet below me.
If I fall, I can't fall far.

The prayers that people pray for me
are the hammock that swaddles and enfolds me
as I sleep suspended over the chasm
between what was and what will be.

The prayers that people pray for me
are the sturdy lace-up hiking boots
with Vibram outsoles that keep me grounded
even when the terrain is treacherous.

The prayers that people pray for me
are the comfort, the warmth, the hope of God
made real in words and images,
and sometimes with no words at all.

I feel it, that people pray for me.
I feel it body, mind and soul.
I feel the peace, I feel the strength.

And I vow to pray for others,
especially those whom no one remembers,
so that they can feel it, too.

Thank you, God, for the power of prayer.
Thank you for the prayers of your people.

Embracing Disruption

The podcaster said that Keith Jarrett
agreed to record the concert
as a warning to future show organizers,
as evidence that disaster happens when he
doesn't get his perfectionist way.

I'd never heard of Keith Jarrett.
I didn't know about the famous Köln Concert.
I wasn't listening to jazz in 1975.
But I know a little bit about perfectionism
and confess to one or two of my own
perfection-fueled passive-aggressive moments.

The recording of that concert, the podcaster said,
A concert played on
> a beat up
> broken down
> rehearsal piano
> that was tinny and thin
> in the upper registers
> and weak in the lower
> with pedals that didn't work,

The recording of that concert
> became the best-selling album in jazz history
> and remains the best-selling solo piano album
> of all time.

Disruption released genius.
Disturbance set creativity free.
Dysfunction made space for something astonishing.

God, set me free in this journey,
 free from perfectionism
 free from trying to control every incident
 free from striving for genius
 free from seeking the astonishing
 free even from focusing on what I can learn from this.
Help me just to let it unfold
And to meet you as it does.

Mourning and Lamentation

Today we reached a horrific benchmark:
One hundred thousand dead from COVID-19
in the United States alone,
a disproportionate number of them persons of color,
laying bare again the racial divide
as clearly as does the killing of black men on city streets.
God, help us.
God, forgive us.

Today there is violence in the streets of this city,
a state of emergency and curfew imposed
as parts of downtown burn and
monuments of confederate generals
become flash points of protest.
God, help us.
God, forgive us.

I feel powerless and so very helpless.
I want to be downtown
as a messenger of peace.
I want to be at the monuments
to support those taking risks
to make their voices heard.
I want to pray with the crowds,
share cups of cold water
and envision together
a world beyond racial division.
God, help us.
God, forgive us.

And I am here, stuck here at home,
immunocompromised and vulnerable.
I can't go out to the crowd at all,
especially in a pandemic.
Now chemo feels brutal and cruel.
I am sick of it, literally,
and sick that it keeps me at home.
God, help me.
God, forgive me.

All I can do (and it is enough) is
pray and pray and pray some more
for your people on every side of these divides,
pray and pray and pray some more
for justice in this city, our nation, our world,
pray and pray and pray some more
knowing that there is power in prayer,
and trusting that prayer is part of the healing.

God, hear our prayer.
Help us to pray what you want us pray
and to ask for what you want to give.

PSALM AGAINST
"At Least"

O God, when they start a sentence with "At least,"
please silence their tongues.
When they want to encourage me with "At least,"
please mute their voices.
> At least they caught it early.
> At least the tumor is small.
> At least they don't do radical mastectomies anymore.
> At least you are healthy and strong.
> At least you're still young.
> At least you've got good insurance.
> At least you know that God is with you.
> At least you'll only have four infusions.
> At least you'll only have sixteen radiation treatments.
At least.
At least.
At least.

I don't want the least.
I don't want the least of any of this.
I don't want the pittance
> the leftovers
> the lowest
> the minimum.
I want the most of life
> and healing
> and grace
> and love.
I claim the most of all that you intend, O God.
Life abundant. Even here. Even now.

So, when they begin their consolations with "At least,"
let me smile kindly,
trust that they intend more,
and claim the most.

PSALM OF
Jesus on the Swirling Wind

The night before chemo
I follow a guided meditation I found on YouTube.
A calming voice invites me to descend a staircase
into relaxation.
I picture the walkway from the top of the
Guggenheim Museum
      spiraling down to the ground floor,
      but it is too crowded.
So, I move to the empty staircase
      under the road to the zoo at Bear Mountain.

On step five, the voice pauses
and invites me to reach out to my spirit guide.
My cry arises quickly and fully,
      without a thought,
      without my conscious intent,
      "Jesus, I need you."

If I'd thought about it
I would have called
      Mary Magdalene
      or the Holy Spirit.
After all, as I began the descent,
the voice invited me to imagine
      wearing a flowing gown
      of whatever color I chose.
      I chose red.

But my cry is to Jesus.
    "I need you."
    And he comes.
    Immediately.

At first, he is unmovable darkness at my left hand,
    a pillar,
    a crag and stronghold,
    a castle to keep me safe.
Stable. Comforting. Present.
    And too, too solid.

I don't speak out loud,
but Jesus hears and becomes a long swirl of thick white silk,
    delicate and substantive at once,
    like the silk scarves I've been dyeing,
    only more luxurious.
Silken Jesus on the wind,
    swirling all around me,
    above me,
    below me,
    beside me,
    at times passing through me
    with the gift of sheer peace.

The voice beckons me to take step six.
Suddenly the red dress feels all wrong
    and I change in the blink of an eye to
    the luxurious heavy-weight
    luminous delicate whiteness of undyed silk.

Jesus and I descend together one step at a time.
When we reach the bottom of the staircase,
the voice invites us to go to a peaceful blue sea.
We go to the Atlantic,
    steely grey water
    and crashing waves,
    my recharging place.

Jesus stays beside me,
    a solid black pillar
    and a flapping, swirling,
    dancing silk on the breeze.
Next to me. Over me. Within me.
St. Patrick's breastplate made real,
    not as solid masculine armor,
    but in a feminine swirl of silk.
    Christ beside me,
    Christ above me,
    Christ beneath me,
    Christ within me.

We go back up the staircase.
Ascending from light to light,
    I fall asleep quickly and soundly,
    safe in Jesus' swirling love.

Jesus on the swirling wind,
    flowing, whirling,
    dancing, twirling.
Pure brightness enfolding,
    leaping, emboldening,
    lighter than air.

Silk on the breeze,
> light beyond all light,
> love beyond all love,
> joy beyond all joy.

You dance at my side.
> You lift me high.
> You reach right through me.

Every molecule of my body
> is known and caressed by your silken love.

Every fear is lifted and carried away.
> Every illness is raised to your own heart.

Jesus on the swirling wind, stay with me.
Dance at my side,
> over me,
> under me,
> in me,
> around me.

Dance me to healing.
Dance me to wholeness.

The First Chemo Infusion

How can this be, O God?
When I thought I would feel afraid,
when I feared I would feel alone,
I am infused with love.

I put on my blue flowered dress this morning,
the one I wear for traveling.
I feel pretty and strong and brave
and ready for an adventure.

I enter the cancer center all alone.
You'd think I would be terrified
doing this at all, no less in a pandemic.
Instead, I feel a warm and calming hope.

My nurse navigator sits with me in the waiting room,
giving me the blessing of her presence.
I'm Chatty Kathy, talking too much and too fast.
(I guess I am a little nervous.)
We chat and sit until I am called in.

I enter the infusion room for the first time.
You'd think I would be terrified.
Instead, I am mostly curious.
My blood pressure is only slightly elevated.

Now I am seated in a recliner
just across from the nurse's station
where they can keep an eye on me
in case of adverse reactions.

My nurse introduces herself.
She tells me she is happy that I have a port.
She explains that if the veins collapse,
as they often do with these particular drugs,
the chemicals seep and damage surrounding tissue.
She says she is thrilled that I will be spared that pain.
For the first time, I'm grateful for my port.

A man in the corner is snoring away.
I almost envy him, except that
I want to be present to all of this.
I don't want to miss a single thing.

My nurse accesses my port
and the drugs start flowing.
Saline, then steroids.
One chemo drug, then the second.
Anti-nausea drugs and more saline.
It will be just over three hours
from start to finish.
I'm tolerating it well, they tell me.
I'm accepting this well.

How can I be so fearless?
How can I feel so loved?
There must be a whole lot of people
praying for me today.

Chemo Blues and Other Colors

PSALM OF
Puppy Love

It occurs to me to wonder
as Tom drives me home from my first chemo infusion—
now that strange fluids flow through my veins,
will Georgia turn up her nose
and avoid me like the plague
the way she did for three days
after I ate homemade Korean fish soup
during a parish visitation?

We arrive home.
I empty my chemo gear bag
and sit in my living room chair.
Georgia comes to me.
She sniffs (uh oh, here it comes)
then asks me to pick her up.
She sits on my lap as long as I sit
and sleeps at my side as long as I sleep
for the next three nights and days.

Praise God for loyal pets
who know what we need
when we need them the most.
Praise God for puppy love.

Dexamethazone

God I feel good
    so good   really good
        so much better than I thought I would   feel
better than I hoped it would be
        than I felt in weeks
       and even the hip that aches all the time
           is not aching at all right now
   at two o'clock in the morning   when
          I'm wide awake and
      sweating through my   pajamas
and better get up and change
    them and I'm so thirsty and   nothing hurts at all and
        I'm happy they were so professional and so
      nice to me during the infusion   and kind and
gentle and it didn't hurt and I had a
     cup   of tea and a little yogurt and I
   drew and wrote in my journal and   prayed
        for the people in the room and asked lots
of questions and wrote
    down
         the answers and didn't feel   lonely going
      into that room alone all by myself because of
       COVID restrictions and   Tom couldn't
   come with me and
even my hip that aches all the time   doesn't
      ache and I can't get my
        rings off because my fingers

are swollen and it didn't   hurt and
            nothing hurts and   I feel

good so good   really good   so
    much better than I thought it would be
            better than I hoped I would feel   right
                now at three o'clock in the morning   and it's
    quiet and lovely and I'm so   thirsty and
        the dog is snoring and Tom is
                        kind of snoring and I better
    change my pajamas again and
I have to go back to the cancer   center
    tomorrow morning for the shot that helps
            something or other that I can't remember right
    now but I'll remember in the morning and
        I'll get there on time and Tom
    will drive me because I don't
            think I should do that   tomorrow
        so I don't even have to worry about
                not sleeping when I feel

good   so good
        really good
    so much better than I thought it   would be
            better than I thought I would feel   even with the
        fullness in my chest and the
                        weirdness in my brain and I'm
    so thirsty   and I don't hurt at all
        at four o'clock in the morning as I
    change my pajamas   for the third time

PSALM OF
The Long Bones

"All my bones shall say, 'O Lord, who is like you?'"
My bones are speaking today. I hear them crying out.

I returned to the cancer center the day after the infusion
    for a shot that stimulates the bone marrow
    to produce white blood cells.
The nurse described everything she was doing,
    bringing the drug to room temperature
    so that it wouldn't be painful,
    injecting it slowly
    so that it wouldn't be painful.
It was not painful.

She told me a little about her life as she worked,
    how a patient gave her the nickname she still goes by
    after years of her own unusual name evoking
    one too many painful jokes
    about a part of the body deemed less honorable.
She told me about the potential side effect of bone pain,
    told me what to do if I suffer it this time,
    and how to mitigate it next time.
"If you get it, it won't last long," she told me.
I walked out the cancer center door just twenty minutes
after arriving.

Now, two days later, my long bones are speaking.
Mild bone aches move from pace to place—
    femur to tibia,
    fibula to metatarsals,

humerus to metacarpals,
to ulna, phalanges, and clavicles,
even to my cheekbones,
although they are not long.
It's not pain, but aches,
like the kind that come with the flu,
making my body think I'm sick.
I tell Tom, "I don't feel well, but I don't feel bad,
especially compared with what I feared."

Praise God for bones that speak
and prove that they are doing what they should.
Praise God that they won't speak
for more than a few days.

Being Recognized

As I am leaving the infusion center,
I hear a voice calling, "Bishop Goff!"
I look around. Who in this place
knows me by that identity?
I look around again.
I don't recognize any of these masked people
in their infusion lounge chairs.
She calls a second time and waves.
She is a member of one of our congregations.
I don't put a name to her half-face until she reminds me.
We chat about my visit to her church last fall.
We scarcely acknowledge chemo.
Respecting COVID distance, I bless her from afar.

I wondered if I might feel too vulnerable,
being seen as patient when I've always been pastor,
but it never occurred to me in the moment.
Instead, it was good to be seen and known from my
other world
and to see the connection of two big pieces of my life
in the eyes of sister chemo traveler.

PSALM FOR
The Temple of the Spirit

My nighttime routine takes longer now.
I rub ointment on my toenails
and slather my feet with thick moisturizer
then pull on clean cotton socks.
I rub ointment on my fingernails
and slather my hands with the same cream
then put on clean cotton gloves,
all to keep my nails and protect my skin.

In the weeks before Mom died,
I tended her nails and feet.
It felt sacramental then.
It feels sacramental now
as I do these things for me.
It is not a burden.
It is not even a chore.
It is tending God's temple.

"Do you not know that your body
is a temple of the Holy Spirit within you?"
I know it now as never before.

PSALM FOR
Losing My Taste

Suddenly I have no taste.
I, who have always prided myself on
    funky and tasteful clothing,
    chunky and tasteful jewelry,
    spunky and tasteful hairdos,
suddenly have no taste at all.

So don't blame me if my coloring is off.
Don't blame me if I choose weird foods.
Don't blame me if I sit when you come in.

Blame it on my tastelessness.

(From permanent loss of taste
and perpetual tastelessness,
good Lord, deliver me.)

PSALM ON
The Worst Chemo Day

My God, my God, O God,
How can I possibly do this
For two more months?

When I'm Like Naaman

I've always been a little amused
And more than a little judgmental
of Naaman.

A commander of an army,
a man in high favor,
suffering from a skin disease.
He goes to the house of the healer Elisha
and asks for a cure.
Elisha sends a note,
"Go, wash in the Jordan seven times,
and your skin will be restored."

And Naaman is angry.
"I thought for me, he would surely come out
and stand and call on the name of the Lord his God
and wave his hand over the spot
and cure the leprosy."
I thought for me.

I thought for me, I confess,
they would respond more quickly.
I thought for me, I acknowledge,
they would make appointments happen sooner.
I thought for me, I admit,
they would care more, say more, do more.
I thought for me.

Naaman's servants call him on his anger.
"If the prophet had commanded you
to do something difficult,
you would have done it."
He listens and immerses himself
seven times in the Jordan
and his flesh is restored
like the flesh of a young boy.

You call me, O God, on my frustration.
My Naaman phase lasts only a short time
before you humble me and wash me over
with a sense of the value of every life.

PSALM OF
The Colors

On the eve of the second infusion,
as I lie in bed in prayer,
I see all the colors of the rainbow
washing over me,
saturating every organ
with waves of healing light—
        the red of connection,
        and orange of creativity,
        the yellow of confidence,
        the green of love,
        the blue of truth,
        the indigo of openness,
        the violet of wisdom.
All the colors of the rainbow
bathe me in awe and calm.

I miss seeing my swirling Jesus on the wind.
I tell him so and hear, as surely as if he spoke the words,
that such experiences don't happen every day.
And it's ok. I know he's here even when I don't feel him.
The wonder of color is wonder enough.

PSALM OF
The Dream of Green

"God makes me lie down in green pastures,
God leads me beside still waters."

Today in the wilderness
of cancer treatment,
I am in the oasis.
In chemo time
I don't remember dreams as before,
but I remember this one.

I am in lush greenness,
a wet, dripping, vibrant place,
rich with life
Hildegard's veriditas—
  lavish,
  lush,
  dense,
  luxurious,
  succulent,
  sumptuous,
  sensuous,
  verdant,
  nourishing,
  healing,
  holy.

I am safe and full of wonder,
peaceful and calm.
I come to life in the dream of green.

A Bigger World

I'm an old hand at this now,
no longer a neophyte in the infusion room.
I'm still asking lots of questions,
still learning and making connections,
but not so anxious.

My world is bigger now than last time
when I could scarcely see beyond myself,
when my universe was not much more
than my own recliner.

This time I am in the whole room,
observing and paying attention.
There are five of us in this quiet corner,
four women and one man.
The woman to the right of me
just finished and will come back tomorrow.
She'll have three infusions over three days.
Soon I'll have a new neighbor.
I am in good company.
We can't talk much
given the distance between us,
but I am not alone.

It is good, dear God,
to be made bigger,
to go wider,
to have huge space
for the experiences of others
alongside my own.
I like my world bigger.

Bald!

PSALM FOR
Cutting My Hair

I cut my hair very short before it starts to fall out.
My hairdresser offers to come
and cut it for me on the back porch.
It feels too risky in a pandemic,
so I thank her and do it myself.
It's not as if it needs to look good!

As I cut, I see whirls and swirls,
the natural lay of the growth around the crown.
The hair on top of my head grows toward the center
and wants to stand straight up,
just like it did in my baby pictures.
And here, for all these years,
I thought Mom slicked it up that way.

I cut my hair short before it starts to fall out.
A sacrifice. A sacrament.
An outward sign of loss that will come
so that healing can be done,
so that your healing, O God, can be done.

The First Signs of Hair Loss

I'm glad I made my "bald is cute" cancer card weeks ago.
I don't feel so cute today.
Last week I cut my hair very short and purpled it up.
For a few days I enjoyed the spiky spunk of it
and held out hope that it wouldn't fall out after all.

And now it has begun. My scalp feels tender and sore.
Clumps of hair come out every time I touch my head.
I knew it would happen.
I didn't know I would feel so sad.
Knowing something is going to happen
doesn't take away the sting when it does.

Hair loss makes this all too real.
I am sad to the point of tears.
With Tom's help, I cut it even shorter.
I rub coconut oil into what is left.
Did I make the right decision?
Will I regret this?

I don't feel so cute today.
Not today, dear God.

PSALM FOR
Losing My Hair

"Even the hairs of your head are all counted."
Even the hairs of my head.

But what about the hairs
that are not on my head?
What about the hairs
In the shower
In the sink
On the bathroom floor?
On my pillow
In my bed
In my dresser drawer?
On the sofa
In my shoes
On my yoga mat?
On my papers
In my books
In my gardening hat?
On my tee shirt
In my mug
In my jewelry box?
On the keyboard
On the desk
In my hiking socks?
On my easel
In my paints
On my prayer chair?

On my husband
On our dog
In my underwear?

Are the hairs still numbered
in the vacuum cleaner bag?
Will I still be yours
when I'm bald?

My Bald Head

My bald head is not so shocking
when I look in the mirror.
Not anymore.
My skull is not as lumpy bumpy as it feels.
It's actually kind of pretty.
I'm not at all embarrassed or ashamed
(there's so much else in the world
that is clamoring for that response).

Tom hardly seems to notice.
Georgia doesn't care in the least.
She sits on my lap, shedding like a fiend.
If it weren't June when she should be shedding,
I'd think she's in sync with me.
Of course, she always is.
It turns out that hardly anything has changed.
The dreaded blow to
my self-image hasn't come.

My bald head is not so shocking anymore.
Instead, it's now a canvas for my
new artistic medium of headscarf wrapping.

God fill me with colorful art.
God fill me with joy in thanksgiving.
God fill me with shocking delight.

PSALM AS
A Head Wrap Rap

I'm not goin' to wear a wig.
No, I'm not goin' to wear a wig.
I'm just like an eagle,
I'm bald, serene, and regal,
And I'm not goin' to wear a wig.

So I'm tyin' on a head wrap
wrapped 'round a skull cap,
an overlappin' cloth cap,
no mishap, no handicap.

I'm bindin' on some cool silk,
smooth and fresh as cold milk,
not the ilk of cornsilk,
you can't bilk me in pure silk.

I'm fastenin' on some cotton,
the fabric I'm not hot in,
of textures fit for knottin',
and colors not forgotten.

I'm wrappin' round the bald pate
a celebratin' first-rate
rejuvenatin' ornate
don't-I-look-great-in wrap.

I'm not goin' to wear a wig.
No, I'm not goin' to wear a wig.
I'm just like an eagle,
I'm bald, serene and regal,
And I'm not goin' to wear a wig.

Journeying On

PSALM ON
A Good Chemo Day

I don't remember what I thought
when I first woke up this morning,
but it wasn't "I'm in cancer treatment"
or "I feel awful"
or "How long, O God?"
It was simply a normal thought for a new day.
If what lies ahead in each cycle is two or three miserable days
with decent-to-good-to-great days on either side,
I can do this.
I can do this, O God.
Help me do this.

The Washing

"The Pharisees do not eat anything
unless they thoroughly wash their hands,
and they do not eat anything from the market
unless they wash it."

Because of chemo I am like a Pharisee.
I wash and wash and wash my hands.
I wash and wash and wash my food.
I wash and wash and Tom does too.

Together we wash
    our eggs before we crack them,
    our fruits before we peel them,
    our fish before we cook them.
We wash and wash and wash,
not to follow regulations,
but to clean away contagion
while I'm most vulnerable.

So picture this,
picture grapes and blueberries,
cherries, apples, plums,
with fish fillets and fresh brown eggs,
    all lounging in a spa,
    all soaking in a pool,
    all washing up for dinner.
No Pharisee would ever picture that!

PSALM OF
The Side Effects

From night sweats
And nightmares
And nights full of restlessness,
Nights when I hardly can sleep,
Good Lord, deliver me.

From bone aches
And headaches
And days full of heaviness,
Days when I just want to weep,
Good Lord, deliver me.

From hair loss
And nail loss
And loss of distinctiveness,
Loss of things I'd rather keep,
Good Lord, deliver me.

From rashes
And itches
And private-parts tenderness,
Blotches of red on each cheek,
Good Lord, deliver me.

Good Lord, deliver me,
Deliver me, please.
Good Lord, now
Give me your peace.

PSALM OF
The Beast

This beast is stealthy.
This beast attacks without warning.
This beast changes tactics in an instant,
coming from different directions,
    all at once,
    relentlessly,
    unmercifully.
When I think it has done its worst,
this beast circles back again—
    and again
    and again.

This chemo beast is so enormous
that it dominates everything
and so minuscule
that it infiltrates follicles and nail beds.

This beast burns and bruises.
This beast buffets and batters.
This beast steals sleep
and ransacks appetite
and depletes my every reserve.

Still, I don't want to kill this beast.
I don't want to befriend it, either.
I just want to send it deep into the forest,
the way St. Francis sent the wolf of Gubbio,
where there is no one it can harm.

I am so sick and tired of this beast
that I am learning its ways.
And knowing its ways,
I can hang on
    and keep going
    and face this beast
    for as long as it takes.

Then may the wilderness
take back the beast
forever.

Going for the Cure

I meet with my oncologist
    between infusions two and three.
I like her more now as I see
    the engaging woman
    with good bedside manner
    who likes what she does.
    (The differences between
    my first impression and now are,
    it's clear, more about me than her.)
She says, "Your numbers are very good".
She says, "Overall, you are doing well."

But she seems alarmed when I show her photos
    of the bottoms of my feet
    mottled blood red and ghostly white.
    It lasted only fifteen minutes each time
    on two different days, I tell her.
    She asks if the skin is peeling.
    I say no.

I ask her what it means.
She names foot and hand syndrome
    (I think hoof and mouth disease
    which is something else entirely),
    an unusual side effect,
    perhaps capillaries breaking
    and allowing the chemo drugs
    to seep out and damage tissue.

My hands were mottled, too, for a short time.
Heat and cold made it worse.

"When we're going for the cure," my oncologist tells me,
"I like to stay the course."
I like the sound of that, going for the cure.
"In this case, I'm going to reduce the Taxotere.
We'll see how that goes and reassess
before your last infusion."

I'm glad we're going for the cure.
I'm mildly worried that the reduction
        will increase the chance of recurrence.
I worry that the mottled effect didn't really happen,
        that somehow, I made it up,
            but I've got the pictures to prove it to myself.

I don't want permanent damage.
I want to keep walking and working
with my hands during treatment.
Overall, I'm good with the change.
I think. I hope. I trust.

God, let me be good with this decision
as we keep going for the cure.

A Third Infusion Eve

I have been in an oasis for a few days now.
Tomorrow it's back to the wilderness.
How do I go back?
The biblical story says the people simply
moved on when the time was right.
I follow their lead and prepare to move on.

I remember wildernesses I have loved—
    the forest of Olympic National Park
    the back country of the Wind River
    the mountains of New Jersey
    the high desert of northern Arizona
    the Burren of Ireland
    the Badlands of South Dakota
    the bush of Kenya
    the back woods of Virginia.
I've hiked in them and camped in them,
    always following a trail map.

I have not loved this chemo wilderness.
There is no trail guide here, no map, no campsites.
I have not loved the wilderness of chemo,
and I'm headed back tomorrow.

Jesus, be my trail in the wilderness.
Be my campsite and resting place.
Show me your wonders.
Give me your love.
Dance me to healing.

PSALM OF
No Worst Things

My nurse navigator visits with me
before the third infusion.
She asks me how I'm doing.
I tell her I'm doing pretty well,
that chemo isn't the worst thing
that's ever happened to me.

And that gets me thinking.
I don't have a list of worst things.
I don't carry one in my head or heart.
I've never made one and
don't want to start one now.

This chemo is real, but cancer still isn't.
I'm not in denial; I am doing this thing,
but I don't see myself in terms of cancer—
not victim, not warrior, not survivor.
I think of myself as on a journey,
or as doing a project, the way Dad
made projects of managing his health.
Cancer will always be part of my story,
but it is not a part of my identity.

I don't have a list of worst things,
and chemo isn't on it.

How Not to Be Afraid

Do not be afraid.
Again and again, I
    read those words in scripture,
    hear them in prayer,
    say them to others.
"Be of good courage,"
I say in blessing at the end of every worship service.
"Do not be afraid, because
    God who created you
    is always with you
    and loves you fiercely."

Do not be afraid.
At first, I hear the words as
    one more task to accomplish,
    one more job to complete,
    one more thing to check off the to-do list.
And I end up feeling like a failure
each time I'm still afraid.

Oh, foolish me.
Oh, frightened me.
Oh, controlling me.

Here's how to let go of fear.
Here's the illogical way,
the counterintuitive way,
to let fear fall away—

Recognize it.
Name it.
Embrace it.

Name fear as the anxious little brother
　　whom big sister faith
　　loves and trains,
　　and from whose frightened antics
　　faith brings light and hope.

Let fear be for a little while,
until it creates tiny fissures
　　in your everyday armor
　　through which God will slip in
　　and land softly on your heart.

Do not be afraid of fear
which, in faith's embrace,
cracks your shell and
breaks you open just enough
for God to slip on in.

PSALM ON
Zoom

Here I am, back at the cancer center
in the infusion room for the third time,
sitting in the comfortable lounge chair,
drugs running through the port in my chest,
not lounging at all,
but on a Zoom call,
planning a conference with colleagues.

What am I doing, God?
Working even here?
I can scarcely pay attention.
I see my friends, which is healing balm,
but because of the activity around me,
I turn off my camera and they can't see me.

What am I doing, God?
Working even here?
I can't really pay attention.
I speak up and add a thought.
My colleagues are quiet. Too quiet.
I realize that my comment had nothing to do with theirs.
I realize that I'm not able to pay attention.
I love my work and love my colleagues,
but am just not with them.
I really don't care about the conference right now.

When my nurse comes to remove
an empty bag of meds and replace it with the next,
I write to my colleagues in chat,
"Thanks, team. I have to sign off now."
And I do before anyone can respond.

What am I doing, God?
Working even here?
Help me balance the ordinary
with the extraordinary,
to work, yes, but not to escape in work,
to stay present to the present, always,
and not miss any of
the little, ordinary gifts of this journey.
Still my workaholic brain, O God.
Calm my trembling soul.

Coming Alive

PSALM OF
Honey Healing

I know your love, O God, in sweet honey healing.
Honey on my lips to soothe the itch.
Honey on my cheeks to keep redness at bay.
A daily facial of honey straight from the jar.
Manuka honey every morning.

A Facebook friend of Tom's, Kirsten
from New Zealand, suggested it.
It's a common complement
to cancer treatment there.
I don't know if I'd have
a rash red chemo face without it,
but I sure don't with it.
So, I continue my routine
every morning.

Sweeter far than honey,
than honey in the comb,
sweeter far than honey
is your healing, O God,
is your sweet,
sweet honey healing.

PSALM OF
Coming Alive

"The glory of God is a human being fully alive."
St. Irenaeus said those words eighteen hundred years ago.
This cancer treatment is bringing me to life.
I've long thought that being fully alive,
being more like Jesus,
would be amazingly wonderful.
Now I know that the cost of coming alive is high.
The cost is high.
There is no going back now,
and I don't much like the way forward.
So how, how, how can I see
the wonders that are here at hand?

I'm up, then down,
then cruising along,
then full of good spirit,
then frustrated and angry
and scared all over again.
I really don't like this,
  this being so vulnerable,
  this being so mortal,
  this beyond-my-control,
  real, messy, painful life.
I liked the illusion of invulnerability better.

Slowly, so very slowly,
I am coming to terms with this.
Slowly, I am accepting
the awful sacrifice of good health now,
for the sake of good health in the future.

Open my eyes, O God.
Open my ears.
Open my heart.
Bring me to life, fully alive.

PSALM FOR
Another Decision Point

I dream that I am ascending a mountain
with a woman I meet on the trail.
We come to a steep wooden ladder.
I start up. She falls behind.
I'm desperate to get to the top,
driven to reach the snow
so that I can plunge my hands into the cold
and stop the burning at last.

I wake up itching and burning from
a rash and hives over more than
fifty percent of my body.
It erupted over the weekend.
I set an appointment to see
my oncologist as soon as
the office opens on Monday.

She says,
> "You won't be able to continue
> the most toxic of the chemo drugs,
> I'll have to switch you to another drug
> for your last infusion,
> You'll have to see a cardiologist
> because that drug can damage the heart."

I ask about the risks and benefits
of not doing the fourth infusion.

She says,
    "There haven't been any studies
    to compare three versus four,
    some of my patients have stopped after three,
    it is your choice and I'll support you either way."

Then my oncologist has another thought
and sends me to a dermatologist
        to determine if the rash is an allergy to the chemo
        and opine whether it is safe for me to continue.
The dermatologist, hugely great with child, says,
    "Yes, it is an allergy to chemo,
    yes, you can continue chemo,
    with the current drugs and the help of steroids."

I feel a flash of anger.
That's not the answer I wanted,
though I don't know what I'd hoped.
A miracle would have served.

What do I do?
Stop now and take my chances?
Or continue on and take my chances?
I don't know how to decide.

Then in prayer, I read these words,
"I am about to do a new thing.
Now it springs forth, do you not perceive it?
I will make a way in the wilderness
and rivers in the desert."

I am near to tears as I read.
God has been making a way in my wilderness,
Do I not perceive it?
Not fully—but, Yes, I do!

And now God is making a way again.
I can almost see it.
"I give water in the wilderness,
rivers in the desert,
to give drink to my people,
the people whom I formed for myself
so that they might declare my praise."

I can make this decision.
Even though new rashes continue to erupt,
even though it itches and burns like hell,
even though I may have the same response next time,
the allergic reaction won't kill me,
the sleepless, sweaty, thirsty
nights on steroids won't, either.

I'll finish this. Because this is the way in the wilderness.
This is the way through the wilderness.
It is not the way I want, but it is the way I've chosen.
And I will do it so that I never have to do it again.

The Brave Dream

I am dreaming every clergy person's nightmare,
fueled by chemo meds. A terrifying combination.
I need to get to the church to do a Sunday visitation.
I don't have a sermon, I haven't read the lessons.
I am not prepared, but I need to go.
I set off walking through darkness, delays, and detours.

As I walk along, I realize that
all I have to do is call an Uber—
it is a legitimate church expense.
I pull out my phone, but it is liquid.
More darkness, delays, and detours.

I keep trying to get to the parish visitation,
totally unprepared but determined.

I grasp one last chance to find out
what the appointed readings are.
I head upstairs to my studio.
It is a long, long staircase.
I start up the escalator.
The place should be empty
but I hear noises upstairs.
I am frightened and fiercely determined.

As I ascend, I hear sounds again.
"Who's there?" I call out in my sleep voice,
all thick-tongued and imprecise.
"Who is it? Tell me. Tell me now."

My sleep voice gets louder,
though not any clearer.
I keep calling and confronting.

Tom calls my name and I wake up.
He says my cries went on
longer than he's ever heard them.
I feel inordinately proud.
I was brave.
I shouted down the terrors.

Now the sky is growing light
as the rain pours down.
Now is a new day, wet and wild.
Last night I was brave.
Today I will be brave.

PSALM OF
Ginger Rogers

There's a saying that Ginger Rogers did
everything Fred Astaire did,
only backwards and in high heels.

I am Ginger Rogers now,
not seeing where I'm going
but stepping lively
as I dance backwards
through dual pandemics
in spike-heeled chemo shoes.

May I be as graceful as Ginger,
as humble, as alive.
May I dance the dance with abandon.

PSALM OF
Jesus' Question

Two blind men cry out to Jesus on the road,
"Have mercy on us."
Jesus turns to them and asks,
"What do you want me to do for you?"

It seems obvious. Of course he knows.
And still he asks, "What do you want me to do for you?"
They say, "Let our eyes be opened."
Jesus, moved by compassion, touches their eyes.
They regain their sight and follow him.

As he asked the blind men, Jesus now asks me,
"What do you want me to do for you?"
Of course he knows. But I don't. Not yet.
So, I sit and listen and write my response.

> I want you to give me strength and grace
>   to endure chemo tiredness.
> I want you to heal me of this cancer forever.
> I want you to make me wise enough to manage
>   three crises at once as I serve your Church.
> I want you to take away my sinful insistence
>   that I have to meet every need
>   that every person brings to me,
>   that I'm not worthy unless I'm
>   working and producing all the time,
>   that I have to be superwoman
>   who can do everything,
>   even during a pandemic and cancer treatment.

I want you to take away my blindness and give me sight
     to see you,
     to depend on you,
     to follow you, and you alone,
     more truly than ever before.

What do I want you to do for me?
Jesus, my Jesus, my silk on the wind,
I want you to dance in me.

The Wisteria

I'd rather have a yard with bamboo
than a yard with wisteria.
Any time. Any place. Any day.
Bamboo I can just kick over
(our last backyard was full of it).
Wisteria requires a bended knee
    and a reaching down
    and a cutting off of new vines
as close to the ground as I can manage.

Wisteria is popping up everywhere now. It's
    in the flower beds and lawn,
    in the stone and gravel paths,
    under the garden shed,
climbing the dogwood, azalea, and fig tree.

I could go out and cut it down today
in the coolish morning of a hot summer day
and it would be the only thing I'd do today.
The one and only thing.
I think I'd rather spend my limited vigor
on painting this vacation day.
Yes, I think I'd rather be painting.

Wisteria, have your way.
Before the summer's over,
your day will come.

Praise God for growing things,
　　　for life that wants to live,
　　　for life that won't give up
　　　today or any day,
for life that just wants to live
and for the choice I have to let it.

The Imposter

God, I feel vulnerable.
God, I feel exposed.
I keep working through treatments,
    leading a community
    through multiple pandemics
    while remaining physically distanced.
It is holy work, healing work, hard work
and sometimes I am washed over with doubt.
Sometimes I feel like an imposter.
The weaker I am, the stronger the feeling.

Imposter syndrome run amok.
Imposter syndrome on steroids.
Imposter syndrome in need of chemotherapy.

I want to embrace again the Alleluia
    of not knowing what to do
    that leads to gathering the right people
    who end up batting it around
    and figuring it out together.
I want to embrace again the try and fail,
try and fail, try and fail
before getting something right.
So, I will. I simply will.

Alleluia. I don't know how to do this.
Come to think of it, none of us do.
None of us have been through a pandemic before.
That means there are no experts.
And if there are no experts, there are no imposters.
And if there are no imposters, then I'm not one.
Not me. Not now. Not anymore.

PSALM OF
Holy Wisdom

In my mediation the night before the last infusion,
I descend the steps and invite Jesus to join me.
He comes silently, so silently.
Just as quietly, another figure joins him.
Head to toe in red,
    fire engine red,
    glossy nail polish red.
I see no face or features, but I know who she is.
Jesus doesn't speak a word, yet tells me,
    "I sent her to represent me,"
    before he steals away.
He didn't have to say her name.
I know who she is—
Sophia, the Holy Wisdom of Christ.

She is silent
as she stands beside me
at the water's edge,
    silent,
    solid,
    strong,
    secure.
In her silence, I hear
    gentle words of hope,
    bold messages of assurance,
    fierce tidings of good courage.
I felt them all when Jesus danced them.
Now I hear them in the wordless stillness.

Praise God for Wisdom so wise
    that she speaks most clearly of all
    in sheer and utter silence.

Praise God for Sophia,
    holy Wisdom of Christ,
    sister, guide,
    standing at my side,
    teacher,
    companion,
    friend.

PSALM FOR
No Ringing Bells

There is a custom, not ancient but common.
Patients ring a bell at the end of their last chemo treatment.
Friends and family come to hear the ringing and to celebrate.
My cancer center shares the custom. They have a bell.

Except, yet once more, the pandemic strikes.
I finish my last treatment to no fanfare at all,
no recognition, no audible outburst of joy.
Damnable coronavirus.

Except, I wonder,
How does the bell sound in the ears
of those whose treatment feels endless?
How does it land on the hearts
of those whose chemo can't cure them?
How does it fall on the souls
of those whose care is palliative only?

If they'd offered a bell for me to ring after my last infusion,
I would have rung it. I like ritual, after all.
On reflection, though, I'm glad they didn't.
I'd never want my joy to cause another person pain.

Instead, I ring bells silently.
I clang gongs and chime chimes
and make singing bowls sing
in the still, quiet and joyful depths of my being.

Not Out of the Woods

PSALM OF
The Sleeping Dog

Four days past the last infusion,
I'm wrung out, feeling clobbered.
Georgia stayed by my side all night,
literally stretched out
full length along my flank,
as close to me as my own skin.

Her warm body told me,
"I know you don't feel well
so I'm going to stay right here with you.
I will not leave your side, no matter what."
And she didn't. Not until I got up
and she curled up in a tight ball
in the indentation left by my head in the pillow
and went back to sleep.

Praise God for staying with me
in the form of a little sleeping dog.
Praise God for reminding me that
I am not alone.

The Old Friend

At four-thirty in the morning,
when the steroids rob my sleep,
I go back to meditation.
I head down the staircase,
relaxing more each step of the way.
I stop as usual and ask my guide to join me.
Jesus? Sophia? No one comes.
I ask again. Still, no one comes.
I don't feel a sense of absence, only curiosity.
This response is new, as every one is new.

I continue down the steps, alone but not lonely,
and end up on the street where I grew up.
I lie down on my back in the fragrant grass.
Karen, my childhood best friend, lies beside me.
Our hands pillow our heads
as we watch the clouds move slowly by.
We say nothing. We just lie there,
no past, no future, just present,
just the way we did when we were kids.

Praise God for Jesus who came after all,
Jesus with me in my friend,
my dear, old, oldest friend.

PSALM OF
The Hurricane

The remnants of a hurricane approach us.
Winds and rain begin to pummel us.
We sit on the back porch to watch,
feel, and hear it all.

The hurricane outside increases just when
the hurricane inside me begins to settle down.
The hurricane outside picks up in earnest just when
the hurricane inside me begins to subside.
The hurricane outside will make the earth greener, just as
the hurricane inside me has greened my heart with hope.

Praise God, you tempestuous winds,
sheering and clipping and pruning the trees.
Praise God, you tumultuous rains,
drenching and quenching and soaking the ground.
Praise God, you turbulent hurricanes,
changing, reforming, reshaping the earth.
Praise God, you storms of every kind,
clearing out and making room for the new.

PSALM OF
Being Changed

As I emerge from the second bout
of body-wide chemo rash,
I remember a dream.

I am a young student at a new university.
Somehow, I find my way through darkness
    that is as smoky as Istanbul on the fall night
    when people light their coal furnaces
    for the first time.
I make my way, without directions
    or signs of any kind, to the music school.
    The students there are secretive,
    insiders in a well-hidden club.
I meet another outsider, another young woman.
    I ask her if she plays an instrument.
    She says no.
    I ask her why she's here.
Before she answers I say,
    "I don't know if you are a person of faith.
    For me as a person of faith
    this being here is no coincidence.
    It is a God-thing. It's a call."
I hear my own words and know that,
    even though I am an outsider,
    even though I am not accepted
    and probably never will be,
    I am called to sing!

I begin in the richest chest voice I can muster:
    "Behold, I tell you a mystery,
    we shall not sleep,
    but we shall all be changed."
I sing the recitative.
    I feel it rumbling
    low and deep in my chest.
    I sing powerfully
    of mystery,
    of change.
I wake from the dream to the sound of my own song.

I am being changed in this wilderness.
I have been changed.
Holy mystery. Holy change.
Praise be to God for holy change.

PSALM OF
The False Returning

Today I cracked some eggs
    without washing them first.
Today I began mentally listing
    which headscarves I will give away.
Today I imagined getting out of the house
    and doing things long deferred—
    having a massage,
    going to the chiropractor,
    seeing friends in person.
Today I was ready to leave the wilderness.

Except, except,
    the pandemic is still raging,
    infections are still increasing,
    people are still dying.
I'm ready to get back out into society
and there is no society to get out into yet.

For now, it might be a good thing.
It is too soon to leave the wilderness
that still has so much to teach me.

PSALM OF
The Sewing Machine

I take out the sewing machine
to make a mask for an ordination service.
Red, of course, from the same fabric
as the red turban I'll wear.

It is not a successful venture.

Between
the shadow of peripheral neuropathy,
chemo nails and chemo brain,
I can't thread the machine.
When I finally do, the stitches are ugly and uneven.
I can hardly hold a needle to do the hand stitching.

I finally complete the task
two hours after beginning.
It is not a mask to be proud of,
but it will get the job done.

Thank you, God, that I am not upset
about the mess I've made of it.
Healing is coming.
I will be able to sew again, if I so choose.
Thank you, God, that for now
a less-than-perfect mask is perfectly OK.

PSALM
Not Out of the Woods

I'm not out of the woods yet.
Chemo is done.
Chemo side effects are dissipating.
I'm ready for radiation.
And I'm not out of the woods yet.

But there is more light in this part of the forest.
There are fewer beasts and biting bugs.
The unpleasant surprises are less frequent.

I'm not out of the woods yet.
And it is good. Because I'm not done yet,
not ready yet to cross over to the promised land
with all its trials, regrets and disappointments.
There are still plenty of wonders to be found right here,
right here in this forest, right here in this wilderness.

God, show me the wonders that still await
in the wildness of this place.
Show me what you still want me to see.

Never Again

I meet with my oncologist three weeks after the last infusion.
    She celebrates that I have completed chemo.
    She says, "I'm counting on never giving you chemo again."

I rejoice. Never again!
And I am aware of the mild reservation—
she's "counting" on it. There are no guarantees.

My blood work shows that I am
no longer immunocompromised.
Thanks be to God.
I can let go of some of the extraordinary precautions—
    no more washing bananas before peeling them—
while holding on to others as the pandemic continues.

My oncologist adds that I can experience
some compromise for as long as a year after chemo,
so I shouldn't go crazy—my word, not hers.
Not to worry—I'm not the going-crazy type.

I'll see her again in three months.
For now, I hold on tight to Never Again.
No more chemo. Never again.
May it be so, God. May it be so.

The Radiant Glow

Radioactive Psalm

I am aglow with your love, O God,
and soon to be more aglow than ever.
I am radiant in your presence, dear God,
and soon to be more radiant than ever.

My appointment with the radiation oncologist is finally set
after days and days of insurance preauthorization glitches.
Radiation is glowing on the near horizon at last.

In preparation, Tom and I watch the movie *Radioactive*
about the life of Marie Salomea Skłodowska Curie
(it seems like the right thing to do).
What a woman!
Strong, ornery, driven, stubborn, brilliant.
The world is changed because of her dedication—
for better and for worse.
Radiation is both gift and curse.
I am grateful for the gift.

The next morning, I sign consent forms,
I have my first CAT scan
and then I get my first tattoos.
A dot right between my breasts, another on my ribs.
They are nothing like the body art I see everywhere,
but they are mine, my very own.

Soon I'll begin treatments that will come
every day for three weeks and a day.
If the schedule holds, I'll complete them
on the Feast of St. Michael and All Angels

and the birthday of my oldest sister, Dyanne.
She braved the wilderness for fourteen years
after being diagnosed with ovarian cancer.
Fourteen years! Completing my treatment
on her birthday will be my tribute to her.

So let the glow begin.
Let the radiance begin.

PSALM OF
Real Life

All this is not a mess to be endured
until COVID and cancer are over
and real life resumes.
This is as real as it gets.
My life is now.
Thanks be to God.

PSALM FOR
Not Helping

"Heaven helps those who help themselves."
Thank God that's not the word of God
who helps us unconditionally,
who helps us for the love of it.

I go to my radiation simulation.
I meet LINAC—the linear accelerator
that I'll come to know well in the next month.

The radiation technicians show me how to get into position,
then they roll me and push me and pull the sheet under me,
lining up lasers with my tattoos.
"Don't try to help," they say.

I didn't know I was trying to help.
Of course, I was trying to help.
I don't know how not to help.
I don't like not helping.
Not helping makes me feel helpless.
I don't like feeling helpless.
"Don't try to help" doesn't help
and it's what I have to do.

Ben Franklin may have been nobody's fool,
but his oft-quoted words are too transactional for me.

Heaven help me to help myself by not helping at all.
Heaven help me to trust God's help when I'm no help at all.

PSALM FOR
Breathing

You are closer to me, O God, than my own breath.
You are closer to me than every breath I breathe.

It is my first radiation treatment.
    I'll remember to breathe.
I try not to help as they get me lined up.
    I'm remembering to breathe.
The technicians tell me not to move.
    I try to remember to breathe.
The technicians leave the room.
    I remind myself to breathe.
I am alone with LINAC as it comes to life.
    I stop breathing. I can't help it.
I tell myself to breathe and not to move.
    I'm afraid that if I breathe, I'll move.
They tell me not to worry
    and just keep breathing,
That the treatment is quick
    but too long for holding my breath.
And still I clutch.
    It is hard to fill my lungs.
I am shaky. I am trembling.
    I am close to tears as I lie still.

This is so easy after chemo.
    I don't feel physical discomfort.

I don't feel a thing
    except naked and exposed and vulnerable.
I guess that's more than enough.

Soon I'll be an old pro at this.
    Soon I'll breathe without even thinking.
For now, I have to remember to keep breathing.
    Just keep breathing.

When Radiation is Easy

Radiation is easy now.
I can breathe the whole way through
    the drive each morning,
    the short wait,
    the removing my headwrap,
    the changing into a gown,
    the getting into position,
    the treatment,
    the getting dressed again,
    the saying "thanks"
    and "see you tomorrow,"
    and driving home again.
It's all a whole lot easier and quicker now.

My skin is a little pink,
    just pink,
    no burn,
    no blisters.
Just a little rosy and a little itchy.
And it's so much easier now.

It would be nice to have friends
accompany me each day.
And I'm OK that the pandemic precludes it.
I'm in the rhythm, in the groove.
It's becoming rote and I'm glad for it.

God keep me present to the present,
    grateful for the grind,
    rejoicing in the rut
    where your healing is happening.
God keep my thanks on track.

PSALM OF
Confidence

Look how amazing I am, O God!
Look how amazing you have made me!
After six months of isolation,
thirty-six weeks of being
at home or at the hospital,
I did a remarkable thing,
    a marvelous thing,
    an extraordinarily ordinary thing:
I stopped at a gas pump
and filled my car with gas!

In COVID time!
In mask and gloves!
Part way through radiation!
I filled my car with gas!

I am the champion of the world!
I am the queen of the universe!
    I am the conqueror!
    the vanquisher!
    the victor!

Yes, dear God, I am inordinately proud of myself.
I've got my mojo back. I've got my confidence back.
I'm as pumped as the gas in my tank!

PSALM OF
The Ordination Services

Four men and four women are presented this week.
    A cluster of clerics.
    A dedication of deacons.
    An oblation of ordinands.
Ready to be made priest.

It is our first in-person worship
since the pandemic began.
    Eight services.
    One ordinand at each.
    Ten people in the room.
    Distanced and masked.
    Live-streamed services.
I feel safe. We are safe
and joyful beyond words.

I wear red chimere,
    Purple ring and earrings,
    Red and purple turban,
    Matching red mask.
They wear black and white
    As canvas for the
    hanging-down-straight
    red stole that will come.

God's faithful. God's beloved.
God's YES men and women
living at the intersection
of compassion, suffering, and joy.

Each service follows the same liturgy
and each one is unique.
Each service invokes the same Spirit
who comes in different ways.
The Spirit shows up. God's work is done.
The Church has eight new priests.

After months at home,
     months in treatment,
     months in pandemic isolation,
I am out. In community. With people.
Being who I'm called to be.
Doing what I'm called to do.
Doing it in person, in the moment, together.
Living at the intersection
of compassion, suffering, and joy.

Eight services in eight days.
     I am exhausted.
     I am lifted.
     I am blessed beyond words
and thankful beyond imagining.

PSALM OF
Perfection

I am plagued by the perfect,
preyed upon by perfectionism.
Always wanting to get it right
even when I have no power,
> no control,
> no capacity to do
> much of anything.
Even in cancer treatment
perfectionism haunts me.
If only I
> eat the right things,
> do the right exercises,
> perform each act perfectly,
then, then, then . . .
I don't ever actually finish the sentence.

And then I hear the words of an ancient prayer
in a brand-new way.

"All things are being brought to their perfection
by him through whom all things were made,
your Son Jesus Christ our Lord."

Brought to *their* perfection.
I never heard the *their* before.
Without it, it sounds like perfection
is something external, one size fits all.

There's only one perfection
and everything is
 subject to it,
 shaped by it,
 intended for it.
Everything is destined for just one end,
one universal, sterile, distant, unattainable perfection.

It's all different, though, with the simple addition of *their*.
Things are bought to *their* perfection.
 Elephants to perfect elephant-ness
 which is different from
 trees to perfect tree-ness
 which is different from
 me to perfect me-ness.
Each thing has its own perfection
and it's only perfect in context.

In this newfound awareness, I rejoice to
"Let the whole world see and know
that things which were cast down
are being raised up,
and things which had grown old
are being made new,
and that all things are being brought to their perfection
by him through whom all things were made,
your Son Jesus Christ our Lord."

The Broken LINAC

Radiation Day Eleven.
I show up on time, as always.
The tech comes to the waiting room
and tells me that LINAC is not working.
I ask if that happens often.
She says "More often than we'd like;
it's an old machine."
The repair technician lives an hour away
and services other cancer centers.
If he comes and gets it fixed today,
they'll call me back.
If not, we'll add a day next week.
Of course I can make that work,
but I'm disappointed to think I won't
finish treatment on my sister's birthday.

I drive home in hope.
I just put the key in the front door
when the phone rings.
LINAC is almost repaired.
They can do my treatment.
I drive back.
Back on schedule.
Back on track.

Thank you, God, for skilled repairers.
Thank you for technicians who respect a wish
that they could have dismissed as petty.
Thank you that I don't miss a day
and that you, O God, don't miss a beat.

Crossing to the Other Side

The Angry Port

I am concerned about my port.
After radiation treatment number twelve,
I go upstairs to the surgeon's office.

The nurse takes one look and says,
"Let me get the nurse practitioner."
She takes one look and says,
"I'm going to get the doctor."
My surgeon comes in and says,
"The port has to come out."
Of course it does.
The skin over it has been tearing and bleeding
as if my body is doing all it can to push the thing out.

My surgeon will remove it in the OR and do a repair.
Soon. As soon as possible after radiation is complete.
In the meantime, I'm on an antibiotic
so that it will be clean for surgery.

I don't want any more surgery. Ever.
And I can't wait for this surgery to happen.

PSALM OF
Restless Sadness

It is the day before my last radiation treatment.
A beautiful warm evening.
Three moonflowers are opening.
There is a light breeze.
The birds are singing.
And I feel restless and sad.

I get the restlessness.
Although I'm tired from radiation and antibiotics,
I'm feeling almost myself. I'm ready for—
but there's little I can do.
I can't even go to the grocery store
until this port is out
and the threat of infection has passed.
I understand the restlessness.

But sadness?
This melancholy sadness?

I think it's end-of-project letdown,
like the restless sadness I felt
after I turned in my master's thesis.
Or the restless sadness I used to feel
after leading Christmas or Easter worship
and I'd want to go back and do it all over again.

Seems like I'm standing on the riverbank,
looking across to the other side,
missing the wilderness,
wanting out and wanting in, both at once.
Wanting to walk with God.
Just wanting to walk with God.

The Last Radiation Treatment

The last day of radiation!
The *last day* at last!
And LINAC is not working again!
A different problem this time,
but this time I know its ways.

So, I don't drive home.
I simply wait at the cancer center.
I sit and read.
I go outside in the misty rain
and retrace the steps I took months ago
    from one building to another,
    across parking lots,
    past COVID tents,
    a wire in my breast
    on my way to the OR.
There are no tents now.
The mass in my breast is gone.
I don't feel the aloneness I felt then.

I go back inside and sit down again.
I talk with Gwyn, sister and caregiver of Victoria
    who is being treated for cervical cancer,
    doing radiation and chemo on the same day.
    Victoria is anxious.
    I tell her the best things about
    my experiences when she asks.

When she goes in for treatment,
Gwyn and I talk about Richard Rohr and Thomas Merton
(as strangers do in cancer center waiting rooms).

I tell her about new podcasts Rohr has done.
I see a light turn on behind her eyes.
Victoria, she says, is having a hard time reading
and podcasts could be perfect. I recommend a few.
It is the first and only conversation I've had
with other patients in the sixteen days of treatment.
It happens only because I am waiting
for LINAC to be repaired.

Victoria and Gwyn leave.
LINAC is working again.
I am called in.
My final radiation treatment!
I breathe the whole way through.
I get up,
get dressed and
Done.
And done.
And done at last.
Tom and I
celebrate with cake.
I am done.
So done.
So blessedly, rejoicingly done.

The Port That Needs to Go

My sore and tender port site is a magnet.
As I was putting on my vestments
for one of the ordination services,
the lapel mic battery pack jumped out
of my pocket and smacked me squarely,
right on the port. I saw stars.
What were the chances of that?
It took ten minutes for the pain to abate.

As I was putting a box of popcorn
on a top shelf at home,
it bumped a box of tea bags which
flew out and smacked me corner first,
right on the port. I saw stars.
What were the chances of that?
You wouldn't think a cardboard box
could hurt so much.

I can't wait until this thing is gone,
this thing that did its job
and served me well
and now just needs to go.

God, I'm feeling the pain of my port.
All your portals are praise.
Mine isn't. Not anymore.
God, it will be gone soon
and then my praise will rise.

Journeying On

"From the wilderness of Sin, the whole congregation
of the Israelites journeyed on in stages."
From the wilderness they journeyed on.
From the wilderness I journey on.

They moved to another camp
and to another problem—no water.
I move from the camp of active cancer treatment
and to . . . what?
Life in their new camp required the improbable
—water from the rock.
What will my new camp require?
What will my next challenge be?

They never moved beyond challenges.
The Promised Land was glorious and beautiful
and it was not all it was cracked up to be.
It wasn't an empty space just waiting for their arrival.
It wasn't flowing with milk and honey.
It was a hard land—still is.

Yet they journeyed on in stages toward that land.
I journey on in stages toward a promised land
of life after cancer treatment.
What will that land be like?
What will be its blessings?
What will be its demands?

God, you are already there.
You will be there when I arrive,
even if it isn't flowing with milk and honey.
Show me how to draw fresh water there.
Show me how to strike water from the rock.

The Port Removal

Praise, O Praise, it's coming out today!
Praise, O Praise, healing is on the way!
And Tom is with me!

Surgery is scheduled for eight in the morning.
We arrive at five-thirty.
Tom is with me.
Tom is with me.
For the very first time,
I don't walk in alone.
Tom is with me.

We meet each member of the team.
I write down their names
to pray for them later in the day.

The surgeon comes in and takes one look at the port.
"It's even angrier now than before. It's got to come out."
He circles it with his magic marker,
a big black O on my wounded chest.

Glo places the IV. Quickly and painlessly.
She's been doing it for forty-one years, she says.
Her experience shows.
"I have no friends," she quips.
"No one wants to see the IV cart coming."
I believe the second line, but not the first.

Tom is with me.
The whole time.
For the first time.
Tom is with me
and it is good.
Did I mention that
Tom is with me?

They take me in for surgery at seven-forty.
I'm asleep before the gurney is out the door.
I hear, see, feel nothing. Nothing at all.

It takes a mere ten minutes.
I wake easily in post op.
The water and crackers taste divine.
A sacrament of thanksgiving.
I'm soon back in the pre-op cubicle.
Tom is not with me.
He's gone to bring the car around.

My nurse says, "I'm a big fan of yours."
While vulnerable, I'm recognized again.
We talk a little about pandemic worship
in the courtyard of her church.
I don't remember much.
I feel fine, just a little unfocused.
She gives me post-op instructions,
the same ones she gave to Tom.
Between the two of us, we'll get it right.
    Eat normally today.
    Rest. Don't drive or
    operate machinery today.
    Don't lift anything over ten pounds

for the next two weeks.
(I'll remember to hold Georgia's leash
in my left hand when we walk.)

At nine-thirty we're home.
I'm safe.
This leg of the journey is finally over.
Tom was with me.
I reimagine
    surgeries with him at my side,
    chemo with him at my side,
    radiation with him at my side.
I paint the memories with one more sparkling,
translucent wash of hope and thanksgiving.

I had cancer.
I am cancer free.
I'm doing all I can
to stay that way.
I am blessed.

And Tom was with me.
Tom was with me.
Tom was there!

PSALM FOR
Being Untethered

The port is gone.
No foreign parts inside me.
Nothing my body wants to expel.
I am
> Untethered,
> Unfettered,
> Unshackled,
> Set free.

Detached from the port, I feel
detached from cancer
and from the curing brutality
of cancer treatment.
> Unchained,
> Unleashed,
> Unbound,
> Set Free.

And strangely unmoored, so strangely unmoored
from the wilderness way,
from the fears and the graces and daily wonders.
I am already forgetting what it felt like.
It is already fading into the past.
I am set free. I am grateful.
And I miss the wilderness.
> How crazy is that?
> How crazy is that, God?
> How crazy is that?

It was as real as life gets.
Keep it real for me now, God,
because I don't ever want
to take you for granted.
I don't ever want to take one
    Awful,
    Awesome,
    Painful,
    Joyful,
    Terrifying,
    Beautiful
moment of life for granted.

Monkey Face

In the bright bathroom light, I see it.
Fine, downy, baby hair
not just above my lip, where it used to be,
but on my forehead, cheeks, and temples.

I look it up online.
It's a thing, a real thing—
gauzy hair in unaccustomed places,
as if the follicles haven't yet
figured out their best strategy
now that they're back in the game.
It will fall out, they say.
It won't last long, they say.
If you shave it or pluck it
it won't grow back, they say.

Monkey Face, some call it.
That makes me laugh.
And God, you know
I need all the laughter
that comes my way.
This is my circus, after all,
and these are my monkeys.

For now, I'll enjoy the fuzz on my face,
trusting that it will fall out,
just as I'll enjoy the fuzz on my head,
trusting that it will grow in.

PSALM OF
Uncovering

Six weeks after chemo, my skull begins to tingle.
Seven weeks after, the finest of hair appears.
Downy. Darling. Like a baby's. I can't stop touching it.

Twelve weeks after, I'm tying on
a gorgeous silk scarf in the morning,
    the one Tom gave me years ago,
    the one I wear when I want to look
    elegant and sassy at the same time.
My fingers are all fumbles.
I can't get the slippery fabric to stay.
What's wrong with me? I've done this dozens of times.
    I used to do it without even looking.
    How can I have lost the touch overnight?
I tie on a cotton scarf instead, and even it keeps slipping.

Then it hits me. I'm done.
Just like that, I'm done with scarves.
I have a little hair, I don't need scarves anymore.
I'm done with them.

So, I pull off the scarf
near the end of a Zoom staff meeting.
    "Bishop, you look badass,"
    a trusted staffer says.
I feel strong. I feel secure.
I feel badass and sassy and ready to rock.

Oh freedom!
Oh grace!
Oh badass, beautiful,
sassy healing
of our badass, beautiful,
sassy God.

PSALM OF
Growing Back Hair

"And now that I am old and gray-headed,
O God, do not forsake me,
till I make known your strength to this generation
and your power to all who are to come."

The hair on my head really is growing back.
There's more white than before
and what's not white is darker than before.
It's salt and pepper. It's thick. It's kind of cute.
And it's starting to curl.

As it grows, the curls get tighter.
I look like Bozo the Clown,
or a 1960s grandma with a really bad perm.
I can almost tolerate the first,
the second is too much.
So I cut off the curls, cut it back
almost to my early badass look.
I like that better.

Now that I have hair so that I can be gray-headed,
stay with me, O God. Stay with me 'til I make known
the miracle of your simple presence.

Looking Back, Looking Forward

The Cancer Cards I Never Played

As I move from the chemo corner
 and from the radiation region of the wilderness,
I find a few chemo cards I haven't yet played.
They are the complaint cards:
> Cantankerous
> Crotchety
> Cranky
> Cross.

I kept saving them for when I really needed them.
That time never came.

God knows I've had my cranky moments.
God knows I've been cross.
And the worst of the worst never came.

Thanks be to God for hopeful cards played
 and grievance cards left unplayed.
Thanks be to God for goodness.

The Diagnostic Mammogram

Everyone was kind. So kind.
And compassionate, quick, and efficient.
They relieved my anxiety
even before it had a chance to kick in
and honored my tender mortality
on another Ash Wednesday.

I go to my scheduled post-surgery follow up.
I see the nurse practitioner
    and tell her about the hardness in my breast.
She does an exam
    and says it's most likely nothing to worry about.
    She says it could be scar tissue.
She asks if the surgeon placed internal radiation
    where the cancer had been.
She says they did that routinely
    until a little more than a year ago.
She says that could lead to a thickening of tissue.
    I say no.
She says the blue dye used during surgery
    can cause a thickening of tissue.

She goes to get the surgeon.
He takes a look and says
    it is most likely nothing to be concerned about,
    but says I should have a mammogram
    as soon as I can.

The nurse practitioner goes across the hall
       to the imaging center
       and sets it up for them to work me in.
       Right then and there. That very morning.
The surgeon says, "This is going to turn out fine."
I believe him and am not nervous at all.
It doesn't occur to me that it could be something.

Next stop—downstairs to registration.
       The usual paperwork. And a co-pay.
I say I've never paid a co-pay for a mammogram before.
The same woman who checked me in
       for appointments last year
says I'll have diagnostic mammograms instead
       of screening mammograms
       for the next five years,
       and they require a co-pay.

Next, it's back upstairs to the imaging center.
       More paperwork.
The woman behind the desk and I talk a bit.
We compare hair color,
       mine with its subtle violet hue,
       hers with red highlights.
We talk about the breast cancer
       that makes us sisters across race.
We talk about the COVID vaccine,
       how she had the second dose yesterday
       and had to leave work early
       because she was feeling bad.
"But I feel fine today."

Next the mammographer takes me back
	for the mammogram.
Two images of each breast in the usual poses,
	then an extra and different image
	of the right breast.
As soon as she finishes,
	she takes me to a small room,
	still in my robe, to wait for the radiologist.
My Gabriel, my messenger of hope, comes.
	He says, "Hello. I've seen you before."
I say, "Yes. Exactly one year ago today
	you told me I had cancer."
He tells me he looked at the images
	and didn't see anything concerning,
	but ordered an ultrasound to be sure.
He says someone will come for me shortly.

A technician takes me back and does the ultrasound.
My Gabriel, my messenger of peace,
	comes in and does a little more.
Finally he says,
	"I don't see anything I'm concerned about.
These are normal post-surgery changes.
	We'll see you in a year."

Glory Hallelujah!
Even if it is Ash Wednesday.
Even if I've given up Hallelujahs for Lent.
Glory Hallelujah!
I hadn't been worried about the hardness in my breast
	after all the reading I'd done,
but a morning of "I don't think there's anything
	to worry about" was worrying.

And it is done.
I head home just a little over
three hours after the appointments began.
Relief. Celebration.
Thanksgiving on a day that is
better than ashes on my forehead
to remind me of my mortality.

A Nine-Month Checkup

Nine months since I finished chemo.
Nine months of healing change.
And here I am, back in the cancer center
For a nine-month checkup.
> Hair growing in? Check.
> Fingernails and toenails growing normally? Check
> Energy and stamina increasing? Check.
> Tolerating long term meds? Sort of.

I walk into the cancer center with trepidation,
more than a little fear and trembling.
So much has happened in this place—
> tests and blood draws,
> infusions and injections,
> kind words and long silences,
> strength-robbing drugs meant to assure health,
> death-dealing drugs meant to give life.

Just entering this place brings it all back.
Cancer center high blood pressure
soaring even higher this time because
on Sunday I met a woman who told me
that her breast cancer has metastasized;
It is back after eleven years.
"That must feel so discouraging," I say.
"Not really," she replies. "I had eleven good years."
Her hair is close-cropped, ready for the falling out.

"How many infusions will you have?"
"I'll be on chemo for the rest of my life."
And my compassion soars along with my blood pressure.
So discouraging. Maybe not for her, but for me.
News that I had cancer is news I never wanted to hear.
News that the cancer has metastasized
is news I never want to hear.

Carrying her story close to my heart,
I walk into the cancer center with trepidation,
until Matt at check-in recognizes me
and calls me by name (How does he do that?)
With his greeting and our casual chat
about short hair, mine and his,
I feel my blood pressure dropping.
It is ok to be here. It is ok.

Bless everyone who is here, O God, for treatment.
Bless everyone who is here, O God, to work.
Bless us who are afraid and us who are relieved
As we have one more checkup.

PSALM OF

The Support Group

At last. At last.
Breast cancer support groups are meeting again.
Online. Via Zoom.
There were no meetings while I was in treatment.
Not even online. The pandemic put the pause to them.
Now they have resumed.
Online. Via Zoom.

I click into a meeting.
My nurse navigator and the social worker are there.
And six sisters in breast cancer.
We are all in different stages of treatment.
We all have different stories.
As I talk and listen,
I recognize that I am feeling more feelings now.
I am feeling feelings about diagnosis and treatment.
I am feeling feelings I didn't feel before when
    it was all taking each step in turn to get through,
    all head down and full speed ahead,
    all take charge, buck up, and "I can do this."

Now I feel the heartache of walking to the hospital alone.
Now I feel my anger that I had to do it,
    even though it was nobody's fault
    as rules changed from day to day
    at the beginning of the pandemic.
Now I feel my fear of change and name my fear of death.
Now with these women who don't try to talk me out of it.

Now at last it starts to sink in.
This really happened.
Cancer really happened.
Cancer treatment really happened.
It was real. Completely, thoroughly, excruciatingly real.

Thank you, God, for truth-telling and truth-listening.
Thank you, God, for people to talk to
without self-censoring.
Thank you, God, for the wisdom of sisters,
this sorority of hope.

PSALM OF
Ten Thousand Miracles

I have passed through the valley of shadows,
through rugged, harsh stretches of wilderness.
I feared no evil, but did fear change and loss,
    and you were with me, O God,
    your rod and staff did comfort me.
Surely goodness and mercy did follow me
and will follow me still, all the days of my life.

I know because I have seen miracles,
    ten thousand wondrous miracles
    of love and kindness,
    hope and healing,
    simplicity and trust.
I have caught astonishing glimpses
    of the realm of God
    in ordinary rainfall
    and birdsong
    and husband love
    and words of strangers.
Ten thousand little miracles,
ten thousand daily gifts,
with tens of thousands more to come.

A Woman Out of the Wild

I've been to the wild, O God.
I've been to the wild as your own child,
exiled and, yes, beguiled.
I exit on the other side, not too defiled,
now reconciled.

I've been undressed, distressed, oppressed,
under house arrest in a wasp's nest
on a stinging, stunning, illness-shunning quest.

I've been stricken and strung-out and stressed.
I've been mashed-down and masked-up and messed.
I've been blistered and blustered and blessed.
Yes, blessed. So blessed. So very blessed.

By healing grace.
By silent space.
By prayer's embrace
and love that lifts but won't
erase my story.

You can take the woman out of the wild,
but can you take the wild out of the woman?
I hope not.
'Cause this reconciled, healing child
needs your wildest wild,
your ever-loving wondrous wildest wild.

Writing Psalms

I look back, O God,
I look back to where it started
and to how you led me
on a path that's clearer now behind me
than it was when still before me.

I look back, O God,
I look back to where we started
and to how you led me
on a road that trails behind me
and still spools out before me.

I look back and write down the most difficult moments
and I'm crabby and fearful, angry again.
Poor Tom bears the brunt of it
in a way he didn't have to
when my world was smaller.
I lay those moments down for good
when I lay the words on paper.

I look back and write down the most wonderful moments
and I'm lighter and hopeful, laughing again.
Sweet Tom shares the joy of it
in a way he always chose to
when my world was smaller.
I lay those moments down for good
when I lay the words on paper.

I look back and write and notice things
I didn't notice then.
I look back and write and link the dots
I didn't see back then.
I look back and write and write until
     the trauma that lived in my bones is released
     the stress that got stuck in my joints is set free
     and the lump in my throat,
     like the lump in my breast,
     is gone for good.

I look back, O God,
and shout your Praise
as surely as if I had
tattooed the word
on my chest.
I look back and praise you
for good.

PSALM OF
Peace

The peace of all peace be yours this day.
Overflowing peace.
Living water to parched souls.
La paz incomprensible de Dios.

Peace and more peace.
Prayers and more prayers.
Hope beyond hope.
La paz del Señor.

"Hope is the thing with feathers
that perches in the soul."
God pour down genuine love and hopefulness
so that the next few months go by easily.

The peace of all peace be yours this day.
Overflowing peace.
Living water to parched souls.
La paz incomprensible de Dios.

God's Spirit is binding us together
and sustaining us.
Cristo renueva tu interior para que
todos vean la gloria de Dios.

We pray for you.
I pray for you.
Ruego a Dios, nuestro padre
que ponga su mano sobre tu dolor.

God heard our prayers.
God hears our prayers.
Seguiremos orando.
Let the healing begin!

The peace of all peace be yours this day.
Overflowing peace.
Living water to parched souls.
La paz incomprensible de Dios.

You've joined the club that no one wanted to join.
It seems like more than any one person
should have to deal with.
I admit to being more than a little angry.

There are sweet,
sweet moments
when we are aware
that there is only God.

Be gentle with yourself.
You are the only you we have.
Relax like a goofy dog asleep on his back
Until you are all better.

The peace of all peace be yours this day.
Overflowing peace.
Living water to parched souls.
La paz incomprensible de Dios

I can sort of see
The Holy Spirit right there
Hovering and blanketing you
With love and courage.

I woke this morning
with you on my heart
and a gentle mystic whispering,
"All shall be well."

Hugs to you.
Virtual hugs
Holding you tight in love.
Waves of healing love.

The peace of all peace be yours this day.
Overflowing peace.
Living water to parched souls.
La paz incomprensible de Dios.

Cancerversary

It's two years now since it all began,
since "cancer" invaded my lexicon.
How shall I mark my cancerversary?
What date shall I set?

The day of the mammogram that proved anything but routine?
The day of the second mammogram and ultrasound?
The day of the biopsy?
First meeting with the surgeon?
First meeting with the medical oncologist?
The day of surgery?
First meeting with the radiation oncologist?
The second opinion about chemo?
The third opinion?
The fourth opinion that I canceled?
The day my port was placed?
The first chemo infusion?
The day my hair fell out?
The second infusion?
The third?
The last?
The days of itching in between?
The first radiation treatment?
The weeks of daily treatments?
The last radiation treatment?
The day the port was removed?
The days of stress and resolve in between?
All the days of beauty and wonder?

How shall I mark my cancerversary?
What date shall I set?
For now, two years from the day it all began,
I begin again to mark them all.

How long, I wonder?
How many years
before the dates are unremarkable?
How long, I wonder,
until I stop marking cancerversaries at all?

Afterward

PSALM FOR
Telling Your Story

You've read these words,
a few of them anyway.
You've dipped into my story,
maybe just ankle deep, maybe all in.
You've witnessed my terrors, my hope,
my journey through the wilderness
and out, at last, on the other side.
We are sisters in this club
that we never wanted to join,
sisters and some brothers, too,
in all the wretchedness and wonder
of human beings in human bodies.

You have a story to tell, too.
You have terror and trust,
worry and hope
as you journey along a path
that others have traveled before,
and that many more will follow.

Tell your story.
Sing out your hope.
Cry out your fear.
Laugh and weep and dance.
Try not to miss a damned thing
so that you won't miss
a blessed thing, either.
Use whatever words you have.

As long as they are yours,
as long as they are true,
they hold healing power.

Because you are precious,
you are beloved,
you are beautiful.
You are the only *you* there is
and your unique and tender story
is the only one that can fill a space
that has stood empty and waiting
for far too long.

Endnotes

The title of this book, The Desert Shall Rejoice, comes from Isaiah 35:1–2a.

> "The wilderness and the dry land shall be glad; the desert shall rejoice and blossom; like the crocus, it shall blossom abundantly and rejoice with joy and shouting."

A MASS IN MY BREAST

Psalm for a Callback, p. 4

> "In a mirror dimly." I Corinthians 13:12

Psalm for the Mass in My Breast, p. 10

> "A feast of rich food filled with marrow." Isaiah 25:6
>
> "A land flowing with milk and honey." Exodus 3:8

TAKING IT IN

Psalm for the Valley of the Shadows, p. 20

> "Though I walk through the valley of the shadow of death, I will fear no evil. For you are with me. Your rod and your staff, they comfort me." Psalm 23:4

Psalm for the Ashes, p. 21

> "Remember that you are dust, and to dust you shall return." From the liturgy for Ash Wednesday in *The Book of Common Prayer* of The Episcopal Church, page 265.

ENTERING THE WILDERNESS

Psalm for the Cancer Patient, p. 78

"I can do all things through Christ who strengthens me." Philippians 4:13

Psalm of the Port, p. 82

"Arise, shine, for your light has come . . . You will call your walls, Salvation, and all your portals, Praise."

A portion for the canticle called The Third Song of Isaiah in *The Book of Common Prayer*, page 87, based on Isaiah 60:1–19

Psalm of God's Silence, p. 83

"I believe in the sun even when it's not shining.
"I believe in love even when I don't feel it.
"I believe in God even when God is silent."
Poem found written on a cellar wall after the liberation of the concentration camp in Cologne, Germany. The author is unknown. The text has been set to music by many composers. My favorite version is *I Believe* by Mark Miller. The translation of the text that I use in the Psalm of God's Silence is the one Mark Miller uses in his beautiful and moving anthem.

"The Spirit intercedes for us with sighs too deep for words." Romans 8:26

Psalm of the Wilderness Walk, p. 87

"Be strong and courageous; do not be frightened or dismayed, for the Lord your God is with you wherever you go." Joshua 1:9

DISRUPTION
Psalm of Holy Disruption, p. 97

" . . . our Savior Jesus Christ, who abolished death and brought life and immortality to light through the Gospel." 2 Timothy 1:10

Psalm for Embracing Disruption, p. 101

Inspired by an episode of the radio show and podcast *Hidden Brain* entitled, *In Praise of Mess: Why Disorder May Be Good for Us*, first aired on November 29, 2016. Host Shankar Vedantam spoke with Tim Hartford, author of *Messy: The Power of Disorder to Transform our Lives.*

Psalm of Jesus on the Swirling Wind, p. 108

"My crag and my stronghold,"
"A castle to keep me safe."
Psalm 31:3 *The Book of Common Prayer* translation.

CHEMO BLUES AND OTHER COLORS
Psalm of the Long Bones, p. 118

"All my bones shall say, 'O Lord, who is like you?'"
Psalm 35:10a

Psalm for the Temple of the Spirit, p. 121

"Do you not know that your body is the temple of the Holy Spirit within you?" I Corinthians 6:19

Psalm for When I'm Like Naaman, p. 124

The story of the healing of Naaman is told in 2 Kings 5.

Psalm of the Dream of Green, p. 127

"God makes me lie down in green pastures, God leads me beside still waters." Psalm 23:2

Veriditas. This word, which literally means "greenness," is woven through the writings of Hildgard of Bingen (1098–1179), a visionary writer, composer, visual artist, medical doctor, philosopher and Benedictine abbess. She uses the word to celebrate freshness, vitality and growth.

BALD!

Psalm for Losing My Hair, p. 135

"Even the hairs of your head are all counted." Luke 12:7

Psalm as a Head Wrap Rap, p. 138

The rhythm of the refrain of this rap is inspired by "I'm Not Throwin' Away My Shot" from *Hamilton,* by Lin-Manuel Miranda.

JOURNEYING ON

Psalm for the Washing, p. 142

"The Pharisees do not eat unless they thoroughly wash their hands, and they do not eat anything from the market unless they wash it." Mark 7:3–4

Psalm of the Beast, p. 144

Legends tell how St. Francis of Assisi (1182–1225) brokered peace between the people of the Italian town of Gubbio and a fierce wolf that attacked its inhabitants. In most versions of the story, Francis tames the wolf and the people of the village care for it for the rest of its life. In my favorite version, Francis convinces the wolf to return to the depths of the forest where it can do no harm to the people – and where they can do no harm to it.

COMING ALIVE
Psalm of Honey Healing, p. 157
> "Sweeter far than honey, than honey in the comb."
> Psalm 19:10

Psalm of Coming Alive, p. 158
> "The glory of God is a human being fully alive."
> Irenaeus (early second century–202 AD), Bishop of
> Lugdunum in Gaul, now Lyon, France. His writings
> helped shape the early development of Christian
> theology. In his discourse, *Against Heresy*, he
> wrote in Latin, *Gloria Dei vivens homo,* frequently
> translated (though some would say mistranslated) as
> "The glory of God is a human being fully alive."

Psalm of Another Decision Point, p. 161
> "I am about to do a new thing. Now it springs forth,
> do you not perceive it? I will make a way in the
> wilderness and rivers in the desert." Isaiah 43:19
>
> "I give water in the wilderness, rivers in the desert, to
> give drink to my people, the people whom I formed
> for myself so that they might declare my praise."
> Isaiah 43:20–21

Psalm of Jesus' Question, p. 166
> The story of Jesus healing the blind men is found in
> Matthew 20:29–34

NOT OUT OF THE WOODS
Psalm of Being Changed, p. 181
> "Behold, I tell you a mystery, we shall not sleep,
> but we shall all be changed in a moment, in the
> twinkling of an eye." I Corinthians 15:51–52, as sung
> in the bass recitative from *The Messiah* by George
> Frederic Handel.

THE RADIANT GLOW
Psalm for Not Helping, p. 192

"Heaven helps those who help themselves." This expression originated in *Aesop's Fables*. Benjamin Franklin popularized it in *Poor Richard's Almanack* during the first half of the eighteenth century. Neither these words nor the version, "God helps those who help themselves," are found in the Bible.

Psalm for Breathing, p. 193

You are closer to me, O God, than my own breath. While inspired by many verses of scripture, these words are not directly found there. Poet Alfred, Lord Tennyson (1809–1892) wrote "Closer is He than breathing, and nearer than hands and feet" in his poem The Higher Pantheism, 1867.

Psalm of Perfection, p. 200

"All things are being brought to their perfection by him through whom all things were made, your Son Jesus Christ our Lord." From the Ordination of a Priest in *The Book of Common Prayer*, page 528.

CROSSING TO THE OTHER SIDE
Psalm of Journeying On, p. 213

"From the wilderness of Sin, the whole congregation of the Israelites journeyed on by stages." Exodus 17:1

Psalm of Growing Back Hair, p. 223

"And now that I am old and gray-headed, O God, do not forsake me, until I make known your strength to this generation and your power to all who are to come." Psalm 71:18

LOOKING BACK, LOOKING FORWARD

Psalm of Ten Thousand Miracles, p. 236

> Based on Psalm 23

Psalm of Peace, p. 240

> This psalm is a verbal collage of messages sent to me
> in English or Spanish during the wilderness journey.
> "Hope is the thing with feathers that perches in the
> soul." Emily Dickinson, poem 254.

> "All shall be well, and all shall be well, and all manner
> of thing shall be well." From *Revelations of Divine
> Love* by Dame Julian of Norwich (c.1343–c. 1416),
> Medieval English mystic.

> Spanish translations:
> *La paz incomprensible de Dios*: The
> incomprehensible peace of God.
> *La paz del Señor*: The peace of the Lord.
> *Cristo renueva tu interior para que todos vean la
> gloria de Dios*: Christ renews your inner self so that
> everyone might see the glory of God.
> *Ruego a Dios, nuestro Padre, que ponga su mano
> sobre tu dolor*: I pray to God, our Father, to put his
> hand over your pain.
> *Seguiremos orando*: We will continue praying.

Acknowledgments

I am grateful to the doctors, nurses, technicians, and staff members at the Sarah Cannon Cancer Institute and the Virginia Cancer Institute in Richmond, Virginia. They gave me the gifts of their time and generous presence. They gave me clear and honest answers, even when I wasn't quite ready to hear them. They gave me hope as they held my extraordinary experiences in the ordinary routines of their daily work. My cancer felt less huge and terrifying when treated with competence and compassion by those who offer treatment day in and day out. Many involved in my care might recognize themselves in these psalms, sometimes through thinly veiled images.

I am especially grateful for my husband, Tom Holliday, who accompanied me on the journey through cancer diagnosis and treatment. While the COVID-19 pandemic meant that he could not be at the hospital for my surgeries or at the cancer centers for chemo or radiation sessions, he was always there for me. He held me tight when I needed holding and let me be when I needed solitude. He was—and is—my rock.

Finally, I give thanks for all who encouraged and supported me in this writing process: for Susan Tilt, my best friend and encourager extraordinaire who heard individual psalms as I wrote them; for my colleague and friend, Jake Owensby, who gave me invaluable early feedback; for Sara Palmer who invited me to read some of these psalms in an adult forum at St. Mary's Episcopal Church in Arlington, Virginia; for the clergy who sat with me outdoors on a bright, windy afternoon at Shrine Mont Retreat Center in Orkney Springs, Virginia, and listened, reflected out loud, and responded as I shared a bit of my story through psalms; for the many friends who pushed me to publish this work after I shared some psalms on social media during Breast Cancer Awareness Month; and for Emily Barrosse, Karen Gulliver, Jocelyn Kwiatkowski, Karen Polaski, and the entire team at Bold Story Press who, like loving doulas, helped me birth this baby.

About the Author

Susan E. Goff is a visual artist, writer, and bishop in The Episcopal Church. In 2012, she became the first woman elected bishop in the Diocese of Virginia. She led the people of the congregations, schools, retirement communities and other organizations through the COVID-19 pandemic while taking her own journey through the wilderness of breast cancer. Susan delights in exploring the intersections between spirituality, nature and the arts, always encouraging others to tell their own stories in words or images. Susan received a Bachelor of Arts degree in psychology from Rutgers University and a Master of Divinity degree from Union Theological Seminary in New York City. She shares a colorful home in Richmond, Virginia, with her husband, Tom Holliday, and their sweet, stubborn chihuahua, Georgia. You can follow Susan on X and Instagram @BishopGoff.

About Bold Story Press

Bold Story Press is a curated, woman-owned hybrid publishing company with a mission of publishing well-written stories by women. If your book is chosen for publication, our team of expert editors and designers will work with you to publish a professionally edited and designed book. Every woman has a story to tell. If you have written yours and want to explore publishing with Bold Story Press, contact us at https://boldstorypress.com.

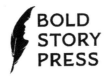

The Bold Story Press logo, designed by Grace Arsenault, was inspired by the nom de plume, or pen name, a sad necessity at one time for female authors who wanted to publish. The woman's face hidden in the quill is the profile of Virginia Woolf, who, in addition to being an early feminist writer, founded and ran her own publishing company, Hogarth Press.

Made in the USA
Middletown, DE
26 October 2024

63322114R00159